Shawnee finds weight loss success after having a baby!

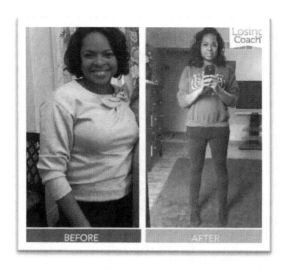

"I began this program with some trepidation as I have tried so many things and failed. I started to struggle with my weight after college and then having a baby and dealing with fibroids, the medications and surgery from it... I was a mess. I was so down on myself because I had been trying to lose weight with no real success and seeing friends who had had a baby and regained their regular bodies back made me feel awful! After learning about Losing Coach and Shelley, I was so willing to give it a try! I love the program! I do not feel shame or judgement about my food choices because the program works regardless of your lifestyle. I also love the daily positive reminders and phone meetings. I have not been doing the program long, but I am proud of the progress I have made thus far. I have gone from a size 8-10 to a size 4 and I am looking forward to reaching my goal by this summer with the help of Losing Coach®!"
- Shawnee

Malisa found her game-changer and lost 64 lbs!

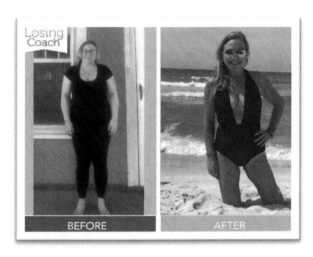

"I was overwhelmed with my weight and how I had let the number on the scale get so high. I dreaded getting up each morning and choosing clothes from the few outfits that still fit—mostly leggings and large tops. How I looked was impacting how I felt about myself, my confidence, and even my ability to allow others to connect with me. I was desperate for help but living in a very small rural community and a random work schedule, that includes traveling, made getting help a challenge. Finding Shelley's online course and virtual support was a game-changer for me. Losing Coach gave me the tools I needed to love and support myself. I could still do so much of what was important to me, like having meals with my family and dining out, while bringing down the number on the scale. Through the encouragement of Shelley and others on their journey, I believe I am worthy of love from myself and others! With 64 pounds down to date, I am lighter physically, stronger mentally and happier spiritually. I love that I have made all my own decisions, which will support me in maintaining the weight loss. Shelley's energy, passion and enthusiasm have helped me realize that the power to change and sustain my health was in me all along."
- Malisa

My Secret Escape

Restore Your Dignity,
Transform Your Body
(it's this way...)

Losing
Coach.®

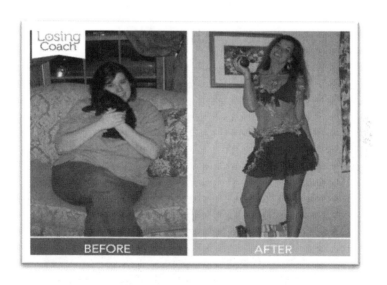

Shelley Johnson
Creator & Founder of Losing Coach

MY SECRET ESCAPE: Restore Your Dignity, Transform Your Body (it's this way. . .) by Shelley Johnson

Copyright © 2018 Shelley Johnson

This book is not intended to be a substitute for the medical advice of a licensed physician. The reader should consult with their doctor in any matters relating to their health.

Cover design by Ellie Searl, Publishista®

ISBN: 9780578411835

First Edition

www.losingcoach.com

GIANT OAK PUBLISHING
Dublin, OH

This book is dedicated to…

My father, THE Bob McDowell (1943-2018). You left me with your brilliant mind, common sense, and integrity to TRUTH.

My kids, as life's greatest teachers, you taught my heart to LOVE.

And ultimately dedicated to my seed of LOVE, the heart, mind and soul of this book

Table of Contents

It's This Way... 1

The Path Out 6

On Your Mark... 8

Weight Gain is Not Your Fault 9

Ignore Diet Industry Advice... 19

The Privacy Principle..................................... 37

One Woman's Weight Loss Journey.............................. 50

Get Set... 69

Accept your Appetite is Real 70

Articulate Your Higher Purpose.. 75

GO!.. 84

The Process from A to Z 85

Steps 1, 2, & 3... 95

Step 1 – POWER.. 99

Step 2 – TRUTH 117

Step 3 – LOVE 124

Step 4 – FAITH.. 134

Step 5 – HOPE 141

Step 6 – SELF CONTROL 154

Step 7 – GRACE 172

Seven Simple Steps.. 182

EPILOGUE 191

ACKNOWLEDGMENTS 193

ABOUT THE AUTHOR.................................... 195

It's This Way...

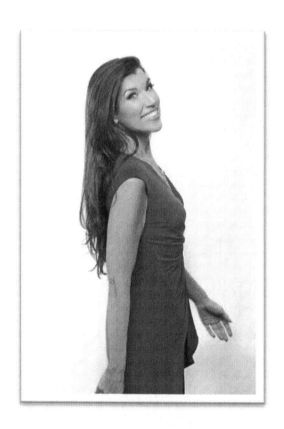

I describe the experience of a woman's weight struggle to a P.O.W. camp. And that is exactly what it is like.

You feel like a prisoner, completely imprisoned and trapped inside a body you can't get out of.

When I was 220 lbs., I intuitively knew that, no way, no how, no matter what I did, right now, at this moment…could I be thin tomorrow.

And it was the overwhelming frustration of that truth that paralyzed me and kept me inside this prison.

But one day, I eventually took *one* leap of faith and got out.

And I'm here to tell you, "It's this way..."

How did I get out?

Honestly, at the time it happened, I had no idea what I was about to do.

That's why it was a real leap of faith.

When you are imprisoned in a prison camp for as long as I was, you really don't know where you are, or what route will lead to freedom.

I knew there were risks and dangers in leaving the camp…I didn't know what was out there, what wild animals would attack, or what storms would hit. I knew I would be completely alone to fend for myself…no guarantee of food, water, or shelter.
I had to trust I would figure it out, *because* I knew that if I stayed, *I would die*.

So, I asked a friend to come with me. She refused.

With or without her, I had to get out.

So, I waited until it was the right time.

When was that?

When I finally reached the end of my rope and realized all hope was lost. No one else was going to rescue me.

My "Will I make it out?" was answered with "You won't make it in here."

All my "but hows?" were answered with "I don't know."

All my "what ifs?" were answered with "Doesn't matter!"

All of my fighting and resistance had ceased. I gave up!

I surrendered.

This is when I could finally make my escape.

And so all alone, secretly and silently in the middle of the night, I crawled beneath the fence to face the darkness alone. It was "*Do or Die!*"

I bolted like a bat out of hell and ran as fast as I could.

I didn't have a clue about where I was going. I didn't know the route in such unfamiliar territory.

I could hear the bullets flying overhead and voices calling me back.

Yet as I continued to keep my eye on the freedom I longed for, pressing forward, and staying low, the clearing got wider.

The voices dimmed. And eventually, darkness turned to light.

I weathered a few storms and survived to make it to complete freedom and safety.

I got out!

Unbeknownst to me at the time, I had found the escape path out of obesity.

Some say I was a pioneer. Some say I got very lucky. Some say it was divinely inspired.

I only know that I got out, and *now*, I *knew the way out*, a safe way out, and I held the map to this escape route.

What happened next paints the picture further.

Erin, an old friend of mine from elementary school, called me. She was amazed at what I had done. She went on and on about it. I could see she was still imprisoned.

So I could only assume she wanted out too, so I asked her if she would like me to help her get out.

Pridefully, she said, "Oh no, I'm fine!"

She had tried so many times before to get out, to no avail, so she had come to accept her imprisonment as her lot in life.

But then I promised her, "I can help you."

See, I absolutely knew that I had found the way out, so I *could* promise her.

She said no again.

But despite her words, I heard *her heart* screaming, "*YES!*"

I touched her hand and said in a very quiet voice, "Trust me, it's this way..."

And simply by hearing my voice say, "Trust me, it's this way..." she too crawled underneath the fence, in the middle of the night, onto the same escape route.

I was there to guide her, to say, "Stay low, the bullets won't hit you."

"Do not pay attention to the voices calling you back."

"Don't worry, the storm will pass."

"The clearing gets wider, and light is coming soon."

So, she followed, and she too found freedom!

She said to me, "Shelley, this is the path to freedom! This is the way! This path is one every woman can take to get out and get out safely. You *have* to go back and help as many women as you can! This is your calling."

I *will* go back for ANY woman who wants out.

Just listen to my voice, "It's this way..."

This is the story of Losing Coach, simply me coaching women on this escape path out of obesity.

The Path Out

The path out. It's this way…

Trapped and lonely, at 220 lbs., I was in despair. I was as desolate as I had ever been. I wanted out, of course I wanted out, but the voices inside the prison were coercing me to stay, telling me I'll never make it out alive. The voices outside the prison were very scary and confusing to me, and they had no idea how trapped I was.

But as I made my escape in the middle of the night and journeyed on this path, I found that I could weather the storms, and as the clearing got wider, I was walking on solid ground.

Not only was it solid, it was fertile! I found myself standing on a luscious field of green and gold by the riverbank.

And on fertile ground, one very powerful seed of LOVE was planted, and a brand-new life was conceived. Like a tree of life.

With time, my roots kept growing stronger and deeper and my branches kept reaching up.

Emerging like a giant oak, I found that as more storms passed, I was still standing. As the years went by, my roots grew deeper and I became stronger.

I was *never* to regain my weight ever again. I now had what I needed for a lifetime. Like a tree of life, one that I hope carries on long after I have left this earth.

I invite you on this path. Hear my voice speaking gently. It's the escape path out. And I will guide you. It's this way…

On Your Mark...

Weight Gain is Not Your Fault

The first thing you need to understand is that your weight gain is not your fault.

Seriously, it is *NOT* your fault!

Your body is simply science.

You have done *nothing* wrong. This is not a character issue. This is not a morality issue. Gaining weight is not your fault!

This is what I teach. You are in this prison through no fault of your own.

And yet, you probably don't believe me right now.

Well I'll tell you exactly why and I'll use science to prove it to you.

Let me explain exactly how your weight gain occurred, and this will show you why it's not your fault. But I don't stop there. I will let you know what you can do about it, how to interrupt this gaining weight cycle in the body, and how to train the brain to stop increasing your appetite.

Understand that I really am talking about science. So, I'm going to explain why weight gain is not your fault, very concisely and very clearly because I know people have a hard time understanding this. I am going to give you a very straight, linear explanation.

First, I'm going to start with an email that I received from a gal from Facebook. She's not a Losing Coach client, she just follows my Facebook and sees the stuff that I post about weight loss and keeping it off and removing the judgement. This is her email:

"Is there some top-secret advice you have for people who can lose a bunch of weight then always lose motivation and start gaining? I lost 40 pounds, then I lost all my weight loss motivation for a few months now and I have gained 15 frickin' pounds back!"

I replied, "Top secret advice? Well, it's not top secret, nor advice. It's an experience you must have. It's the removal of judgement off yourself. Understand that your weight gain is not your fault. It really isn't. I promise you, it's not your fault!"

But women always ask me, "How can you say it's not my fault? That's really nice to hear, Shelley, and it gives me all the warm fuzzies and all, and that's wonderful, but come on, how can you say my weight gain is not my fault? Look at me! Clearly, I've made some poor choices. I know what I did, I know! I know the times that I overate and made bad choices and everything I did. You're crazy!"

I will tell you why your weight gain is not your fault. You are free to argue with me all day long, I will never change my mind. I stand 100% solid on this truth because again, your body is science.

Everyone likes to think they're unique. Everyone likes to think their body is "different". And really, though *this* may be hard to hear, your body is no exception to this rule. It's not, okay?

We're going to start with the weight gain and we're going to work backwards. So, you gained weight...

Gained Weight

Why did that happen? Real simple here, you created a caloric surplus over time. Bottom line. 100% truth, or you would not have gained weight. (Science)

The only way to gain weight is from a caloric surplus. Scientific truth. So, over time you created a caloric surplus.

Gained Weight
↑
Caloric Surplus

How did you create a caloric surplus? Well, you probably ate more. Just a wild guess there. I don't know, just wildly guessing that you ate a little more, over time.

Gained Weight
↑
Caloric Surplus
↑
Ate More

Why did that happen? Most likely, unless you were force fed, it was because your appetite increased.

Gained Weight
↑
Caloric Surplus
↑
Ate More
↑
Increased Appetite

Increased appetite, right? Appetite is defined simply as your desire for food (for whatever reason). So, if you ate more, you desired more food: you had an increased appetite. Well, why did you have an increased appetite?

Your brain did that! You were simply following your brain's instruction. This desire to eat more was an instruction from the brain.

> Gained Weight
> ↑
> Caloric Surplus
> ↑
> Ate More
> ↑
> Increased Appetite
> ↑
> Brain

Okay? Your brain did that! You do not control your appetite, your brain does.

One little quick example. One week I had the stomach flu; I didn't eat anything, because I didn't have an appetite. Didn't wanna eat anything. My brain turned *off* my appetite. I was even *hungry*! But I still didn't *want* to eat anything! Hungry or not, your appetite is defined as your desire to eat food, and your brain controls it!

Okay? Your brain controls your appetite. But *why, why did your brain increase your appetite*?

That is the question! Why would your brain do that? Well again, your body, which includes your brain, is science. And see, it's this complex system of neurology which involves the hypothalamus and amygdala that processes feelings and memories, that affect the appetite. I'm not a neurologist, but I sure wish I was! I have a friend that's a neurologist and she could provide all these technical terms. This is a whole system in the brain that controls the appetite. It's the function of the brain, to ensure your survival.

Okay, so *why* did your brain increase your appetite?

Basically, if your appetite is increased, it did that as a response to that complex neurological system from processing a *feeling* or two.

Gained Weight
↑
Caloric Surplus
↑
Ate More
↑
Increased Appetite
↑
Brain Response
↑
Feeling

Whatever that feeling is. Maybe it's pain. It could be physical pain, or it could be emotional pain. It could be fatigue or tiredness. It could be hurt, anger, sadness, feeling unloved, stress. Whatever that feeling is, physical or emotional, but I'll sum it all up as *anxiety*. Some kind of feeling of anxiety.

Gained Weight
↑
Caloric Surplus
↑
Ate More
↑
Increased Appetite

↑
Brain Response
↑
Feeling - Anxiety

Whether you're in pain, you're hurt, you're angry, tired, or stressed, it's all some form of anxiety you're experiencing.

The brain responded to that anxiety by increasing the appetite. Why? Because the brain knows things from past experiences. The brain likes patterns, and it knows food will decrease your anxiety. Food is a sedative that decreases anxiety, it just does.

Remember when you were a baby and crying and the bottle or the breast calmed you down? You may not, but the brain does. The brain loves patterns, especially the pathway of least resistance (the pathway that's been tread down the most), and one it knows very well is that food eases the *feeling* of anxiety.

So, you had some kind of feeling, some kind of anxiety.

Well, what was that a result of? Aren't you responsible for your own feelings?

Nope.

See, feelings are involuntary reactions. You had an involuntary reaction. Just like if you get punched in the stomach, you will feel pain, an involuntary reaction to the experience of being punched in the stomach. This applies to all feelings, whether physical or emotional., all feelings are involuntary reactions (We'll talk more about that later).

Gained Weight
↑
Caloric Surplus
↑

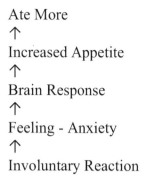

Ate More
↑
Increased Appetite
↑
Brain Response
↑
Feeling - Anxiety
↑
Involuntary Reaction

Where did that involuntary reaction come from? An *experience*.

That's the bottom line here. Maybe that experience was some kind of major life transition, someone mistreated you, someone abused you, you got hurt, you hurt yourself, you got injured, etc. Some way, somehow, you had an experience that created the involuntary reaction of anxiety. Physically or emotionally, you got injured from an experience.

Gained Weight
↑
 Caloric Surplus
↑
Ate More
↑
Increased Appetite
↑
Brain Response
↑
Feeling - Anxiety
↑
Involuntary Reaction
↑
Experience

And whatever experiences you've had, also not your fault. You can't control all of these experiences that happen outside of you. You can't stop those experiences in life from happening. I call them arrows. And I'm telling you, the arrows are gonna keep coming. You can't stop them.

So now you see how your weight gain occurred. Very clearly it is not your fault. Because you don't control your appetite, your brain does. And all of your feelings are involuntary reactions to your experiences.

So, I know now you're saying, "Well, Shelley, then what can I do? How can I intercept this vicious cycle? What can I change? Where can I help myself?"

Well first, I'll tell you where we're *not* going to intercept this cycle. We're not going to try to fight your appetite. And the reason we don't try to fight your appetite is because, the more you try to fight it... You know what happens. You know that fight, "Ugh! I'm hungry! I wanna eat more! But no, I can't eat more! Oh my God, the refrigerator's just calling my name, but I can't! I can't, I can't, I can't!" And the more you try to fight that increased appetite, you're gonna experience more anxiety!

Trying to fight the appetite creates more anxiety, which will only increase your appetite! We've all experienced that, right? The more I say no, the more I want it. So, we're not going to try to intercept there. Once the appetite's increased, it's increased. All you can do is accept it.

What we're going to do in this process, where my weight loss process intercepts this weight gain cycle, is with training the brain. Again, you don't control your appetite, your brain does. So that is what we must do, *train* the *brain*.

So, here's where we intercept - before the brain responds by increasing the appetite, we're going to learn to *accept* all of

these involuntary reactions, these feelings that you have, so they don't increase your anxiety.

Acceptance. That's how we will train the brain. And we're gonna talk about accepting those feelings and decreasing the anxiety that you may have about those feelings from your experiences. We're going to decrease the anxiety and train the brain.

We will be training the brain and healing the heart to intercept this cycle of weight gain that is not your fault. We're going to get you out.

I hope that answers that question once and for all as to why your weight gain is not your fault. But not only that, I will be answering your question as to what we're going to do about it.

Because I was in this prison camp—this cycle of gaining weight through no fault of my own and I couldn't get out. I was imprisoned.

There was no walking out the front door, no asking for a pardon and no one was going to rescue me.

I realized I needed another option.

Escape became my only option. A true, heroic, leap of faith type of escape. Do or die!

And I *had* to escape this prison. It wasn't my fault I was trapped inside a body that would keep gaining and gaining weight, and it would have, if I didn't escape and run for my life!

I'll show you the path step by step. And I've included worksheets to help you reinforce the steps for yourself.

Get ready to run for your life!

Weight Gain Is Not Your Fault Worksheet

Please be specific and as descriptive as you can.

1. A word or two that describes how I feel right now:

2. My weight today:

3. My body is simply _____.

4. Why did you gain weight?

5. How did it happen?

6. Is this your fault?

7. Where can you intercept the cycle of gaining weight?

8. Are you ready to make your escape?

Do you feel like you need personal, inspirational, non-judgmental support from Shelley? Join Shelley's Club now. She can help. It's this way... www.losingcoach.com

Ignore Diet Industry Advice

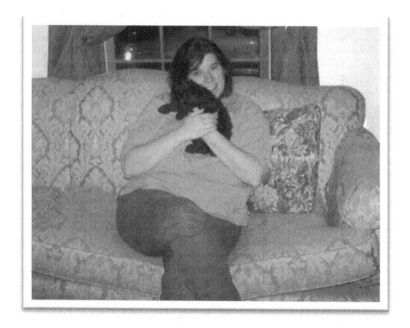

S ee that woman in the photo? That's ME, Shelley. At 220 pounds. I know how you feel right now. Just how I felt in this photo.

A little insecure and uncertain, but mostly overwhelmed. You just feel overwhelmed.

You *are* overwhelmed...with all the "eat this" and "eat that", "don't do this" and "don't do that."

All of the diet industry advice, from what you should eat, to how often you should eat, to what combination of food you should eat has left you wondering what to do and where to start.

I need to remove this confusion immediately. You feel trapped and we need to get you out, so you can take your first step forward.

I started by doing this one thing, and it's simple. You're going to do the same thing.

This is the beginning of *your* weight loss success! Read on to find out about how and why ignoring diet industry advice will help you lose weight and then complete the Ignore Diet Industry Advice Worksheet.

Do ONE Thing to Lose Weight NOW
(Or Really, The One Thing You Should Never Do if You Want to Lose Weight)

I talk with a group of women who are following, know, and have had success with the Losing Coach Process about the one thing they should never do when they want to lose weight.

I do a role-playing exercise with my friend, Erin, to demonstrate how overwhelming the enormous amount of information on weight loss is to most women. Read on to see how I make sense of the absurdity of trying all this conflicting stuff and keeping it up for the rest of your life.

I have a simple, effective alternative for you, it's this way…

~~*~*~*~*~*

Shelley: The one thing you should never do… is listen to *this*! (Holding up piece of paper)

Now I did get this from very reliable sources—a couple of posts on Facebook! (laughing)

This is what you hear out there, I've just compiled it.

Erin: Ok, should I get some paper out?

Shelley: Please, take some notes. You ready?

Erin: I am.

Shelley: How to Lose Weight…

Don't worry about your calories! And make sure you're eating enough! Eat every two to three hours and pay attention to fat. Be sure to eat the right kind of fat! You need fatty essential acids – not the bad fat.

Erin (frantically taking notes): What's bad fat?

Shelley: I don't know, just listen. The trans-fat and saturated fat...

Erin: Eat that?

Shelley: Cut that shit out. (laughing)

Shelley: Give up sugar, alcohol, dairy, red meat, white flour, wheat – that equals inflammation; gluten—that causes bloating, I think that's about the same thing—I don't know. Now, eat only...

Erin: There's still something left to eat?

Shelley: Yes, eat only 4 ounces of lean protein, fish, egg, legumes (leg-oooms, is that how you pronounce it?), beans, and raw or steamed veggies at meals.

Erin, looking confused: Are you going to have a list for me to take home? A menu—something? I mean, this is a lot.

Shelley: (ignoring Erin) IF you eat carbs (laughing) choose low glycemic sweet potatoes, brown rice, etcetera, but go easy on those. No soda, pop, Coke, no matter how you say it, none of that! And, if you can, eat six smaller meals per day, spaced out. Eat lots of fruits and veggies, organic, of course, alkalized with greens.

Erin: How do you alkalize something? Is that legal?

Shelley: Yeah, your body, I don't know, *alkalizes*. So, alkalize with greens, like salads with olive oil, and lemon, seafood, soy products, non-GMO. Ah, this is very important—Drink half your body weight, in ounces, of water, with lemon squeezed in a day! (pause for group mental math) You can figure that out. (chuckling)

Erin: How many ounces?

Shelley: Half your body weight. In ounces. Of water. With lemon. Squeezed. In a day. Also, eat right for your type!

Erin: My blood type?

Shelley: Yes, it's based on blood types, and how foods breakdown, or don't breakdown, and support your body based on your type. And, get moving!

Erin: Yes! I heard that.

Shelley: Do all of this for a month. Your cravings go down. You gain energy, and you feel so much better. And then, keep going. Keep doing all of this... for the rest of your life.

Erin, after a deep breath: Does that work? (women laughing)

Shelley: You tell me. [to the audience] Does this work?

Women from around the room: No! No! No!

Erin, looking out at the women: Have you tried this to lose weight? (heads nodding yes)

Shelley: You've heard all of this, haven't you? It's crazy! Which ones have you bought into?

Erin: I tried the blood type one. [in her best caveman voice] I'm a meat-eater! I'm a carnivore! O-positive. (laughing from the room) Lotsa meat! Wow, that was really heavy. A lot of meat, I mean *a lot* of meat.

Shelley: I used to think it was about the water. I can eat this and that as long as I go drink my water. I am drinking my eight, eight-ounce glasses of water today, so I can eat whatever I want!

Erin: Yeah, I got rid of everything white. That was so intense. Organic, did all that…very intense. Not happy memories for my kids' childhoods. (laughing from the room)

Shelley: Which other ones did you do?

Erin: Well, I remember when I was a kid, my parents did the beet diet. [to the room] Did you ever do the beet diet where you had to eat the beets? You got a half a cup of ice cream. Every day. That was a big deal. We all sat around the table, watching my Dad scoop out a half a cup of ice cream. (laughing from the room)

Shelley: I did a coaching session with someone recently and we talked about the decades—what you were told to do in each decade. In the 1970's it was count your calories. In the 1980's it was cut out sugar. In the 1990's it was cut out fat. In the 2000's it was cut out the carbs. What would it be now? It's cut out all the non-organic.

Erin: Yeah, non-GMO and all that, right? No gluten. Nothing processed.

A participant: The raw diet.

Another participant: And now they're saying cholesterol is not that bad for you.

Erin: Right, now it's coming all back around. Don't even worry about cholesterol anymore!

Another woman: Exercise. You can have whatever you want as long as you exercise.

Erin: Have you all bought into that? I did. It didn't work. So why doesn't all this work?

Shelley: All these diets, why don't they work? It's not that these don't work, or that they're not good advice, but... how can you do it? Eating everything—and nothing? All at the same time. It's literally impossible. It's impossible to worry about all of this. It's like, you just can't keep track of everything that's going on here.

Erin: What does it make people feel like?

Shelley: Like "I can't do this!" This is impossible! Overwhelmed. It is that feeling of "I've got so much to worry about" and you can't even get started then because you're worried about too many things. And literally, I've got to analyze all of this for twenty minutes before I can make a decision about what to eat to see if it fits into this "Do this, don't do that. Eat this, don't eat that." Am I eating six small meals a day, every two to three hours? Oh my gosh, it's been too many hours, I've screwed up my metabolism now, I might as well just quit.

Erin: Yeah, have you tried to do it in the midst of your job? In the midst of going to school? In the midst of kids, in the midst of parents, in the midst of paying bills... to add one more thing to your plate? No pun intended. That overwhelmed feeling. Do you still feel that way? Do you still sometimes go "oh my gosh, I'm so overwhelmed"? When it comes to your weight... Is that a predominant feeling?

Participant: Not any more. Now I only have one thing to worry about. It's journaling what I eat and making sure it falls under a certain calorie amount at the end of the day. And I don't have to spend an hour and a half every night prepping six meals for the following day. Making a grocery list of all the special things, specialty food items I have to buy. I don't have to do that. I don't have to think about that. I just do my journal.

Shelley: I have to say (pointing to the participant who just spoke) she's a doctor, so she's a perfect one to ask. She's not keeping track of any of *this*! (holding up paper she just read from)

(To physician): You're not concerning yourself with any of that. You are manipulating the math by counting the calories and bringing your weight down. Are you now healthier than you were thirty pounds ago?

Physician/Participant: Tremendously, yes.

Shelley: But you're not worried about any of this other stuff? Shutting down your metabolism? Eating every two to three hours? As a doctor, are you concerned?

Physician: Nope.

Shelley: We talked about this the other day, I asked, "Now, your patients when they go in to get prepped for surgery, aren't allowed to eat, right? They're fasting before they go in for surgery. Are you concerned about their metabolism shutting down?"

Physician: Absolutely not.

Erin: Are you concerned about them going into starvation mode?

Physician: Definitely not.

Erin: Are you concerned about them screwing up their metabolism for their future?

Physician: No, not at all.

Shelley: I mean, they didn't eat every two to three hours, six smaller meals, and their health will be okay?

Physician/Participant: Yes, and despite that, I felt like I needed to eat every two to three hours to keep my metabolism up, because that knowledge didn't apply to me. (laughing)

Erin: So, Shelley, you were saying, the one thing you should not do...

Shelley: Is listen to this (holding up the diet industry advice she had read to the group).

Erin: So, you're saying ignore the advice out there?

Shelley: Yes, ignore all the advice out there! Know what you know to be true! Each and every one of you in this room has lost weight with this process, by trusting what you know to be true with the caloric deficit, and that's the only way to manipulate your weight, is through math. You know when you've held on to that truth, what has happened. So, the evidence speaks for itself!

When all of this information comes out on Facebook, on Twitter, in the New York Times; understand that every time that information comes in, your brain takes it in, and you will emotionally begin to feel confused. It's emotional, not rational. Your brain is taking all that in. You feel overwhelmed. The anxiety increases, and you're left feeling confused. So, the one thing you should do if you want to lose weight is <u>ignore everything</u>. And as soon as you see a magazine article, a clip on TV, something on the radio, a talk show, people talking at work, about weight loss, immediately turn it off and walk away. This is the path out.

Erin to Shelley: What do you see regularly with clients when they get confused? What happens to them?

Shelley: Well, they can't even take a step forward. They're feeling trapped in fear. Oh no, what if I don't eat breakfast? I've heard I can't skip breakfast! They're scared of these things they have been told over and over again. Like, they *must* eat breakfast! Listen, I eat breakfast every day. Sometimes it's at noon. The fear doesn't come into me that I'm going to screw anything up with my body. I manage my weight and I'm healthy. I check with my doctor very frequently because I'm a hypochondriac. (laughing) But I'm very healthy! (more laughing)

Erin: So, what is the one thing you should do if you want to lose weight?

Shelley: Truth. Know the truth. Believe in the truth. Believe in the math. You've all already experienced it. But you do need reminded of it because we all get carried away. We hear something, and we consider it for a split second. We think maybe they're right. And naturally, we want to better ourselves, we want to help ourselves. So, when I hear that something is healthy, I want to listen to it. But just keep that separate from the math.

The math is the only thing that is going to bring your weight down. Manipulate that math and create a caloric deficit. Just keep it all separate. Understand that what you do for your health is for your health. What you do for your fitness is for your fitness. And what you do for your weight is math.

Shelley to the group: What have you experienced with ignoring the advice and focusing on the truth?

Participant: I have found it to be very freeing. In the workplace, whenever there are multiple women together talking about the diet they're trying, the competition they're in with each other, or how frustrated they are that something isn't working for them, that they've tried over and over again… It's very freeing just to be able to disconnect from that and walk away from it. And that has really been profound to me.

Shelley: It's like having a secret inside of you!

Participant: Yes!

Shelley: To be able to stand on your own two feet. I can know things, and I can believe things and I can feel things inside of me, and I don't have to prove it to anyone else in this room. How powerful is that?

Participant: It's very powerful. It's a whole new level of confidence in yourself and in your abilities. And a peace, a peacefulness within yourself, and that's priceless.

Another participant: For me it's been freeing because of not having to tell someone when I decide I'm going to lose weight. When I decide to lose weight, I just simply decide to lose weight and I know how to do it.

I have a co-worker who I've told "if you want to lose weight, do not tell anyone, just keep it to yourself."

In a meeting she announced "I'm going to lose weight. I'm going to be sexy this summer. It's my goal for the summer." She's put it out to everyone. So, week after week she'll tell me she goes to the Weight Watcher meetings, each week, and she's not losing any weight, and she feels disappointed. And because she announced it in front of everyone at the meeting and didn't pay attention to anything I said about keeping it quiet, she feels humiliated.

You don't have to feel that way. Keep it private. It's no-one's business, it's no-one's body but your own. For me that's freeing. When I decide to lose weight, I just simply follow the process and that's it. If I decide I want to take a break, that's fine too, but nobody needs to know about it.

Shelley: Isn't it amazing?! Keeping it private. Women find it hard because we're trained in full disclosure. Women find that very challenging to keep it to themselves. Look what it's cost your co-worker. She's embarrassed now.

Erin: So, the one thing you shouldn't do is listen to anybody else about your body?

Shelley: Yes, IGNORE DIET INDUSTRY ADVICE!

~~*~*~*~*~*

When I turned my back on all of this diet industry advice, I started trusting myself and focused on the one truth of losing weight. And then, I lost weight.

That's the bottom line. Here I am, 90 lbs. less, as living proof.

And I'm not different than you. I don't have anything unique that you lack.

I only FOCUSED on the TRUTH about weight loss (Step 2 - TRUTH).

It can be difficult for some to believe that all I did was focus on the simple truth. They have tried to debate this with me and tell me that weight loss is more than math and very complicated. But I will never debate TRUTH, it doesn't need debated, so my only rebuttal is to hold up my Before & After photos and say:

"It's okay, you don't have to believe me." ;)

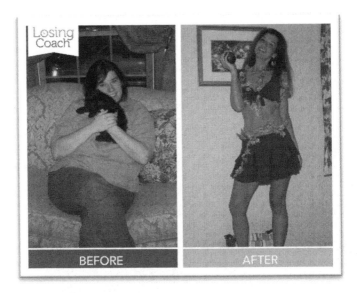

And so, the voices inside the prison, telling me I'd never make it out alive, to the voices outside the prison complicating it, telling me to go in all sorts of different directions, they all became silent.

I silenced them. I refused to listen to anyone any more.

The voices outside the prison had no idea what it was like being inside the prison. And the voices inside the prison were there themselves because they did not know how to get out!

So, nobody's voice had a voice resonated with me anymore, except my own.

Here's to your escape! It's this way…

Ignore Diet Industry Advice Worksheet

Please be specific and as descriptive as you can.

1. A word or two that describes how I feel right now:

2. My weight today:

3. The advice from the diet industry that overwhelms me:

4. Other things I have heard to help me lose weight:

5. The programs and the things I have tried:

6. What has confused me or didn't work for me:

7. What really worked for me authentically:

8. I am throwing out all of these pieces of diet industry advice from now on:

You can get personal, inspirational, non-judgmental support from Shelley by joining Shelley's Club. She can help. It's this way... www.losingcoach.com

Comedy Break: What if Alcohol Treatment Centers Acted Like the Weight Loss Industry

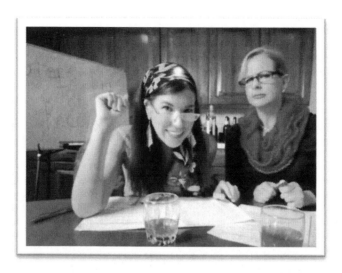

Erin: *Welcome to our rehab center where we help alcoholics like you recover from their alcoholism.*

Shelley: *According to your intake form, you drink too much!*

Erin: *So that makes you an alcoholic.*

Shelley: *If you didn't drink so much, you wouldn't be, but since you do, you've come to the right place and to the right people! Because we are both recovered alcoholics!*

Erin: *If we can do it, anyone can do it!*

Shelley: *So, listen carefully, we've taken all the good advice from the diet industry and created your treatment plan using all of their principles.*

Erin: Because they seem to work. I mean, they are successful businesses, right? A multibillion- dollar industry.

Shelley: So, pay attention. If you want to overcome your alcoholism, do all of these things. First things first, you must start out each and every day with a good strong drink.

Erin: Don't skip that drink!

Shelley: You're gonna want to skip that drink, but trust us, don't skip it. It is the most important drink of the day!

Erin: It is the most important drink of the day!

Shelley: Trust us. We start out each and every day with a good strong drink, don't we?

Erin: Every single day!

Shelley: After that, it's important to continue to drink every two to three hours, but a small drink and stop there.

Erin: It's very important that you continue to drink. We want to keep that buzz going. We don't want you craving alcohol. Make sure you're also drinking six small drinks a day. Remember, just a little bit and stop there.

Shelley: We found that's not too difficult for alcoholics to do.

Erin: Oh, and we want to make sure that you're drinking from all of the alcoholic groups and combining them correctly. Don't neglect any of the major alcohol groups and make sure you're mixing the lean stuff with the more complex choices.

Shelley: Light beer, mixed drinks!

Erin: Top shelf stuff!

Shelley: Champagne, wine...
Erin: Liqueur.

Shelley: We know this is very complicated, but that's okay. We're gonna help you out. We created a pyramid.

Erin: Even the government uses it!

Shelley: It's very helpful, but it is subject to change of course.

Erin: Don't worry about that. We've made it really pretty and colorful, highlighting all of the beautiful choices of alcohol that you have. Hard stuff at the top, your basic wheat beers at the bottom.

Shelley: If you want to watch your drinking, you can attend our support group. Every week we're gonna test your blood alcohol level. If it's down at all, we're gonna give you a gold star!

Erin: If you don't want to pay any attention to what you're doing during your recovery, we can sell you portion controlled drinks for an entire week. Truth be told, it doesn't matter how you do it as long as you come to us for your recovery in any one of these ways for your unexplainable obsession with alcohol.

Shelley: Once you're recovered, it's very important for you to continue to drink in a healthy, balanced way every day for the rest of your life, just like us!

Erin: Every single day!

Shelley: And if all this sounds too complicated, don't worry. We have pills you can take. Oh, they're not addictive. Besides, you don't seem like the type that would have an addiction problem anyway.

Erin: *Right! And if for some odd, unexplainable reason none of this works, come back because we'll need to run some tests. Your blood type, genetics, hormonal and physiological factors that are preventing you from your recovery but... didn't seem to affect us at all in ours. But we'll be here to help you because we're going to be in business for a very long time!*

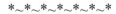

Absurd, isn't it? But this is what you've been faced with every time you've tried to lose weight. Every day you've struggled with your weight. No wonder you haven't been able to lose weight in the past! It's not your fault.

The Privacy Principle

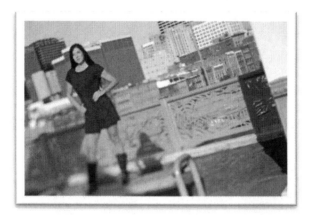

W hen I began my weight loss, I said to myself: "I want this time to be different. I want it to work. And I want it to last. So, it must be *different.*"

And I knew if I wanted it to be different, I must *do* something different.

So I decided to keep it private.

I decided not to tell anyone what I was doing. I decided to not talk about it. I wasn't going to talk about my fat, my body, the scale, or food. I was literally going to keep my mouth shut, about *everything*!

That was different!

In this day and age of social media, "full disclosure", and over-sharing we have been conditioned to share too many things with too many people.

To keep it private, imagine yourself in this photo—in a powerful stance, with your back against the world, your hands on your hips, and your mouth shut.

When I decided to keep it private, it was a simple, yet very magical principle that helped me lose weight immediately. After putting it into practice, I discovered it gave me five things:

1. It Prevents Judgement
2. It Provides Blessings
3. It Propels Self-Discipline
4. It Problem-Solves
5. It Protects Power

Keep reading to find out how the Privacy Principle works and then complete the Privacy Principle Worksheet.

The Privacy Principle

In this Losing Coach session, I talk with a client about the very powerful Privacy Principle.

~~*~*~*~*~*

Shelley: There are five sub-principles to my Privacy Principle.

The first one is it <u>prevents judgement</u>.

I. PREVENTS JUDGEMENT

You know that every time you start a diet program and you mention anything about your desire to lose weight, or your attempt to try something new, or do this, or do that, you know what your loved ones are going to say! They love you very much, but chances are someone's going to make a judgmental comment. It might be a mom or a sister or a friend, and it can be the simplest little comment of them saying, "Oh, let me know how long *this time* lasts!"

You immediately open yourself up for judgement and criticism when you share it with your loved ones. So that's the first point to the Privacy Principle, it prevents judgement from coming your way when you keep it private.

That's what we're here to do, we are here to protect you from the judgement. The first thing that we do in this coaching, is remove the judgement, and after that, we need to protect you from more judgement. So, stay private.

The second thing that privacy does is it <u>provides blessings</u>.

II. PROVIDES BLESSINGS

My Grandpa Bennett used to be the chef of the family. He would have all the family over on Sunday afternoons. He would grill chicken and bratwursts and, of course, his famous potato salad. And he was a big food pusher! You know the type, the food pushers! He wanted everyone to come over and eat and eat and eat!

So, I would go over there and get my plate of food with my appropriate portions and I would eat. Grandpa didn't know I was trying to lose weight since I was keeping it private. His natural thing to say was "Come on, Shelley, eat more! Eat more, Shelley, eat more!"

So, I asked myself, "what does Grandpa want?" Does he really want me to eat more and gain weight? I don't think so! I think the only thing Grandpa wanted is validation that his cooking is delicious. So, I thought, I can give him that validation, verbally. So, I simply said to him, "Grandpa, this is delicious! Grandpa, this is the best chicken I've ever had! Best potato salad in the world. Grandpa, like always!" I would give him that validation verbally and not tell him that I was on a diet. In doing so, he would stop food-pushing, and I provided him with blessings.

And think about this. If I had told Grandpa, "I can't eat anymore because I'm on a diet", or "I'm watching my weight." What have I done? I have now put him on the spot to respond to that statement, that I'm trying to lose weight. Do you know what a spot that puts people on? He has one of two ways to reply.

He could say, "you don't need to worry about that." Well, now I've made him a *liar* because that's a lie. I did need to worry about my weight, but I put him on the spot to tell me I didn't need to worry about that.

The other choice he has is to say, "Good, Shelley, I agree." Well, now I've made him a *jerk*!

Every time that you put someone on the spot to reply to your weight/body concerns, you make them either a *liar* or a *jerk*! Think about that. *A liar or a jerk*! These are the only 2 options a person has when you put them on the spot to reply to any kind of "I'm on a diet" statement.

So, you provide blessings to everyone around you by keeping it private.

Client: I always wondered why every time I said to someone, "I'm on a diet," or "I'm watching what I'm eating," it felt like there was anxiety around what I was passing on to them. They're put on the spot. There are two outcomes, and neither are good.

Shelley: Right! Neither are good. And yes, you're passing it onto them because you've now given them your problem. This is my problem, and now I'm going to make it yours!

Client: It's a big burden.

Shelley (nodding): It's a big burden to people for them to take on your problems. When I tell them I'm watching my weight, I'm on a diet, they just naturally take that on as their problem and then seek to "fix" it, so of course they say, "you don't need to worry about that", which again makes them a liar.

It provides blessings to everyone around you to keep it private.

III. PROPELS SELF-DISCIPLINE

It propels self-discipline. I want you to think about this. You're going to go out there with friends, or your mother-in-law, or sister, and they're all talking. Talk, talk, talk about their diets and their weight, and this food, and that food, and their exercise, and their workout routine, and they're all talk, talk, talk, talk! You are going to be tempted to jump into that conversation. But you're going to think to yourself, Shelley told me to keep it private, so I'm going to bite my tongue.

And then you're out with friends again. Talk, talk, talk, talk, talk! And you're going to think about it and bite your tongue again.

I want you to think about this. Every time that you exercise self-discipline in keeping your mouth shut, guess what you're doing? You're *cultivating self-discipline* to *keep your mouth shut*!

This is the Privacy Principle. You apply the principle in one area of your life. I'm going to bite my tongue (figuratively), I'm going to exercise self-discipline in keeping my mouth shut. It translates into the power of *self-discipline to keep your mouth shut* (literally)! Trust me. I don't know why or how this works, but it translates into the power to keep your mouth shut! It propels self-discipline to keep it private!

Client: It's amazing!

Shelley: Yes, it's amazing. When I tell women to keep it private, they say, "I think that's something I can do. I mean, you're not asking me not to eat the foods I love. Keep it private? Okay, I think I can do that!"

It can be more challenging than they realize, but they can do it! They are propelling their own self-discipline in their decisions with food and in how much they eat because they have trained themselves to have the self-discipline to keep their mouth shut. It's an amazing thing. All you do is follow the privacy principle and you will be cultivating and growing that self-discipline!

IV. PROBLEM-SOLVES

When you keep it private, you enable your brain to problem-solve for you. Understand that your brain is a *natural problem-*

solver. Without you even having to say "solve a problem for me" your brain naturally wants to solve problems for you. That's what it is there for.

I'll just give you a silly example. My boobs are saggy. That's a problem. Okay? It's a big problem. (laughing)

So, the first thing that my brain does to help me solve my problem is it *thinks* about it. I'm going to think about my problem! Okay, my boobs are too low. Maybe I should think about another problem for this, but it's a funny one (more laughing).

Thinking about it is the first stage of problem-solving.

There are Three Stages of Problem-Solving in the brain:

1. Think about it
2. Talk about it
3. Take action

Stage 1 - *Think* about it. This is a valid stage of problem solving. First you need to think about your problem. Isn't this an obvious one?

First, simply *think*. This is when you're *engaging the data*. Okay, I'm looking in the mirror and I'm seeing that they're lower. I'm putting on my bra and it just doesn't fit the same. I am thinking about my problem. But you know what, at the end of the day, my problem still exists. As much as I've thought about it, my boobs are still saggy.

And at the end of the day, even though your problem still exists, your brain actually feels very satisfied that it has helped you solve your problem. It says "check, I've helped you solve your problem!" Because it has, it's been *thinking* about it (that's the first stage of problem solving). So, at the end of the day your brain feels very satisfied, *but* your problem still exists! My boobs are still saggy no matter how much I think about it.

Stage 2- *Talk* about it. The second stage of problem solving is to talk about it. Your brain says "now talk about this" because now you need to collect some feedback. When you talk about it, you are engaging feedback. "Well, you know, I read on the internet, there are three different types of incisions you can get... Which incision did you get? What doctor did you go to? How much did it cost you? Were you happy with the results?"

Now I am *engaging the feedback*. But at the end of the day, my boobs are still saggy, as much as I've talked about it. And again, the brain is very satisfied that it has helped you solve your problem. It says "check. I've helped you solve your problem today" because you talked about it. You engaged the feedback.

There's a time and a place for thinking about your problem and for talking about your problem, because you're engaging the data and you're engaging the feedback.

Stage 3 – *Take action*! When you're done engaging the data, "I've thought about it enough and my problem's still here" and when you're done engaging the feedback, "I've talked about it enough, but my problem's still here" then finally the brain is ready to take action!

"I know what incision I'm getting, I know what doctor I'm going to, I know how much it's going to cost, and I know what kind of results to expect from it." Now I can take action, because I'm done thinking and I'm done talking about it. This is when you are *engaging* the *solution*.

How many people do you know that just talk on and on and on and on about the same problem that they had last week, last year, year after year after year? And you're like. "would you shut up already and do something about it!" Right?

I always say, when you're done thinking about your weight, when you're done *talking*—when you're done collecting feedback from everything and everyone else about your diet, your weight, and *your* body, then you're ready to act!

But you need to be done thinking about it and you need to be done talking about it first to allow the brain to move into that third stage of problem solving—take action.

Client: That's one of my favorites. For the longest time I've thought about it so much. I've made so many plans for this. I'm exhausted just thinking about all the ideas that I have. Why can't I make it happen? Why can't I put it into action? I'm so focused on thinking about it and even talking about it. All these grandiose ideas of weight loss.

Shelley: I know, and people actually get stuck there. But when they are forced to stay private about it, for whatever reason, (maybe because they're listening to me) and they say, "Okay, I'm going to do what Shelley says, I'm going to stay private about it", their brain has no outlet to solve their problem in stage two. It says, "Oh, you're not going to talk about it anymore? Well, I've got to do *something* to help you solve your problem!"

The brain will naturally move from the second stage into that third stage of problem solving and it will enable you to act. Because when you stay private about it and you refuse to talk about it anymore, this will frustrate the brain enough to be like *"OKAY! Do something about this!"*

When you stop talking about it, your brain will naturally move into the third stage of problem-solving by *acting* for you! This *engages the solution*.

The Stages of Problem-Solving and what it does for solving your problem:

1. Think About it - Engages the Data
2. Talk About it - Engages the Feedback
3. Take Action - Engages the Solution

Practice the Privacy Principle by keeping everything 100% private and you will experience all of this ability to take action and engage the solution! It's magical! It works!

V. PROTECTS POWER

The last thing the Privacy Principle does is it <u>protects your power</u>.

You know your weight loss is not going to come from some ingenious system or program you're trying to follow, that it's not the information, but it's about "how do I take this information and find the *power* within myself to put into practice the very thing I long to do?"

That's what people are looking for when it comes to weight loss —the *power* to put into practice the very thing you long to do. Women discover they have this power in the workshop or in the first coaching session. Through step one, this power is inside of them to do it. They're simply not aware of it yet. They have to experience that. Then they realize "I *do* have the power to do this!"

When you stay private about it, you protect this power. If you go and speak about it, you're giving some of that away to everyone who asks you, "What are you doing? What about your weight loss plan? How's your diet?" When you talk about it, you're giving away some of your power that you have inside of you that belongs to only you. Every time you speak about it, you dilute your power. It's like a drip. You start to give it away to whoever wants to talk about your weight and your diet. Protect it. It's no one else's business.

To recap, the Privacy Principle, keeping it private, does five things for you:

1. Prevents judgement
2. Provides blessings
3. Propels self-discipline
4. Problem-solves
5. Protects your power

So, keep it very, very private. It is NO ONE else's business what you do with your body!

Not even a little bit of "oh, I can't have that." As soon as you say, "I can't have that", what have you implied?

Yep, "I'm on a diet!"

It's those very little, subtle, two or three-word phrases that we're used to saying. So, lock and key privacy. Lock and key! It is absolutely nobody else's business what you're doing or why you're doing it.

~~*~*~*~*

And so, in privacy, in complete secrecy, in the black of night, I crawled underneath the prison fence. Nobody saw me. Nobody knew. Because I didn't tell a soul. I didn't make a peep. I crawled underneath to the other side of the fence, onto a path that would lead me to a luscious field of green and gold by the riverbank.

I just had to keep it private and not tell anyone what I was doing. Those on the inside certainly would call me back. Those on the outside would trip me up. I had to do it in complete secrecy in the dark.

But—I got out.

Again, this book is not intended to be a substitute for the medical advice of a licensed physician. The reader should consult with her doctor in any matters relating to her health. Feel free to discuss this process with your physician. It's a one-time breech of the privacy principle that won't hurt your efforts. Physicians love my process! Tell them about it!

The Privacy Principle Worksheet

Please be as specific and as descriptive as you can.

1. A word or two that describes how I feel right now:

2. My weight today:

3. Is "Keeping it Private" a new idea or thought for you?

4. What do you like about "Keeping it Private"?

5. What part of "Keeping it Private" will be easy for you?

6. What part will be more challenging and why?

7. What does "Keeping it Private" mean to you?

8. List ways you can respect your privacy and which sub-principle it provides for you (prevents judgement, provides blessings, propels self-discipline, problem-solves, or protects your power).

You won't need Shelley forever, but she can get you where you want to go while you're learning the process. It's this way...
www.losingcoach.com

One Woman's Weight Loss Journey

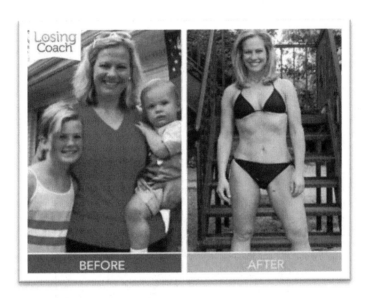

W hen Erin decided to lose weight, she created a video log of her journey with the Losing Coach®.

Experience her powerful transformation right along with her and receive inspiration and motivation from her success.

Feel yourself relating to her thoughts, feelings, and fears as she shares real, honest and raw moments from her journey.

You will see this mother of four transform herself to who she always wanted to be—a glorious, confident and beautiful woman.

Read about Erin's journey and then use the Weight Loss Journey Worksheet to record your own thoughts, feelings, hopes and fears about your weight loss journey.

Erin's Weight Loss Journey

After Erin's hesitation and fear, she took a leap of faith and hired me to help her lose weight.

<u>Day One</u>

Erin: "Okay, so this is day one of my personal transformation journey of taking myself down 60 pounds in weight. I've hired Shelley Johnson to get me there. I'm now at 179 pounds.

I got on the scale first thing this morning; my goal is 120 pounds. My goal is, a year from now, to be able to sit here in front of this blog and weigh 120 pounds. Shelley has assured me that it is completely doable, and she has every confidence in making that happen with me.

She told me, "Erin, that's so easy. We can do this. I promise you, I can help you do this. I promise you."

And I trust Shelley. I haven't been in the 120 range since I was in middle school, which is kind of funny because that's when I first met Shelley. Shelley and I have grown up together, I trust Shelley. I was with her when she was her frumpy self. We've been frumpy girls together, and I know what she was before she transformed herself, so I have no hesitation in entrusting myself to her because she resonates with me and I resonate with her. I know that she's transformed herself and it's real because I've been with her since she was in middle school. So, my goal is to vlog this and see my own progression and just record and chronicle that. Shelley has given me my assignments, I started them this morning. I've started my journal, and she told me to take a before picture which I will do today.

I also decided that I wanted to take a before video, and I'm gonna go ahead and do that. I'm gonna stand up, try to get as much of a full body view as I possibly can and take it from there. Okay.

So, this is me, day one, 179 pounds. There you have it. All right, I'll see you tomorrow."

Day Three

"Okay, so day three of my weight loss transformation. Being coached by Shelley Johnson, the Losing Coach! And I'm down two pounds! I got on the scale this morning, I'm at 177. Very exciting to me to start seeing my numbers going down.

In fact, the excitement of getting on the scale this morning is what got me out of bed. And Shelley told me that I could look forward to getting on the scale every day. She told me to anticipate those numbers going down and she's been right all along. Shelley has been great on this journey as she has continued to encourage me and help me stay focused.

In fact, yesterday I had to go to the grocery store. I was a little nervous about that because I was a little hungry. It was getting to be dinnertime and that was the only time I had during the day to get over there, and I needed to really keep my focus and keep my goals straight in the front of my mind. And lo and behold, I kid you not, Shelley called me while I was in the middle of being at the grocery store. She had no idea that that's where I was, but she wanted to call, see how I was doing, see how I was feeling physically and emotionally about the goals that I had set, and about the assignments that she had given me.

Shelley is very focused with her clients on having them own the entire process. She tells them that this is their assignment, these are their goals. These are not rules that she has established, because they're not. She's helping me make my own goals and establish my own rules and it's empowering. She wanted to know if I was doing okay with that, if they felt right, if I was getting into a groove with them, and that really helped me stay focused at the grocery store.

Because here she was talking with me about my goals. So, that didn't surprise me because that's the way Shelley is, she's very perceptive about what's going on with her clients, even if she's not meeting with them face-to-face directly. She's very aware of them, she's thinking about them throughout her day, and is very in tune with where they are, so it didn't surprise me that she would call while I was there, because that's the way she rolls. So, today is another day. I did a great job meeting my goals for yesterday. I am very excited.

Again, very empowered, and here's another day. You can hear the baby in the background, so this is all real. Onward and upward. So, I'll see you tomorrow. Thanks for checking in."

<u>One Week</u>

"It's been a week since I started my weight loss journey with Shelley Johnson, and I've lost three pounds. I met with Shelley yesterday and she told me that was worthy of a celebration, so we went ahead and celebrated. The thing that I'm most grateful for right now is that I went ahead and made the call to Shelley more than a week and a half ago and told her about my weight loss goals.

I had actually been putting off contacting Shelley for over three months because I was very nervous that she was going to tell me what I could and couldn't eat, and I really was not interested in one more person telling me how to live my life. But that's not how Shelley works. In fact, from my perspective, Shelley is rather revolutionary in the way she approaches weight loss. Contacting her was one of the smartest moves I've made so far this year. I'm really glad that I did, and I'm excited about what the future holds. So, more to come. I'll talk to you tomorrow. Have a great day."

Day 11

I'm at the end of day 11 in my weight loss transformation journey and I have lost about four and a half pounds. The thing that has been very inspiring to me over the last few days is that it's becoming rather habitual to be able to focus on my goals and keep them at the forefront of my mind. And to be able to actually lead my body. I feel very empowered to not only have the tools that Shelley has given me, but to be able to use them for my own well-being, and that's inspiring to me. I don't feel that this is drudgery, I don't feel that I'm deprived. I feel in control and empowered by this process, and that is very inspiring. So, onward and upward. Blessings on you in your endeavors, and may you know the joy and fulfillment that comes from self-discipline."

Day 25

"Day 25 in my weight loss journey with Shelley Johnson. I'm down about eight pounds. Yesterday my husband said to me, "I mean this in the nicest way, but your jeans look really sloppy on you." Yay! So, my jeans are actually too big for me. My weight does seem to be stuck right now, but Shelley told me to anticipate that, so I'm not discouraged because I'm staying disciplined with my goals and my personal assignments. I'm taking my weight loss at a process of four pounds at a time. I figure if I can lose four pounds then I can lose the next four pounds, and the next four pounds. And I've already lost twice as much as that, so I know that this is very doable and that's a manageable means for me to attain my final goal. So, onward and upward with Shelley. She continues to be a real encouragement to me."

Day 33

Erin: Here we are on day 33. I've lost 9.6 pounds.

Shelley: 9.6 pounds in 33 days. You were concerned last week. You told me that you thought you were at a standstill.

Erin: I did, I felt like my weight was going up. I was afraid that it was going up, I was very nervous.

Shelley: And?

Erin: And it didn't. I lost a pound this week, so good.

Shelley: What created that fear? Why were you concerned it was at a standstill?

Erin: Because I had integrated some new things. I had started working out and actually moved back into old thinking patterns. "I really, really have to work. I really have to suffer. This really has to be hard, this really has to be painful." Because I felt that it had been too easy, and I was enjoying it too much.

And then when I talked to you and told you I was afraid of my weight going up, and that "I'm even working out, and I'm being so diligent."

And you said, "But, are you enjoying it?"

And I said, "No."

Shelley: So, you had some kind of pre-programming that you thought you had to suffer?

Erin: Yeah, I did. I totally thought I had to suffer, it had to be hard, it had to be painful. And so, because the previous 30-some days had been so easy and have been so fun, I thought, "That's not right. I can't do that." And so, I saw that old patterns were coming back into play.

Shelley: And so, were you able to kind of release yourself from thinking that you had to suffer?

Erin: Yeah. You sat down and talked to me and I still get chills when I see you and I hear your voice.

You said, "*Don't you think you've suffered enough?*"

And that was huge. That was everything.

(crying) Yeah, I've suffered enough, I don't need to suffer anymore.

And so, I stepped back into enjoying it… and I love who I am, and I love what I'm capable of doing. And you told me that I had the right to enjoy it and so I did, and my body said, "Now, we can get back into this. We can do this, we don't have to suffer anymore." So, yeah.

Shelley: You've lost almost 10 pounds!

Erin: Almost 10 pounds, and I know I have the right to this. And I know I can do this, and you keep reminding me, "You're doing it. You are doing it."

Shelley: Yeah.

Erin: The weight has been a barrier to keep people out, and to keep the real me from being available to be judged, really.

Shelley: Yes, being available to be known. To be seen.

Erin: To be seen.

Shelley: It truly is. And actually, I've described it like this before. Weight is like a blanket. It shields you from the world, from people, from whatever. Openness and connectedness. So, if we have these layers and layers of blankets on, we're protected. So, you've got a jacket on, take it off! (Shelley and Erin both take off their jackets)

Shelley: It's one layer. Okay? It's one layer. All of a sudden, we're a little bit more open, we're a little bit more vulnerable.

Erin: Right, I'm a little bit more exposed.

Shelley: A little bit more exposed. Right. And it's actually good that this weight loss takes time because you are peeling off layer by layer, and with each layer that you peel off, you're opening yourself up to people and the world a little bit more, and you have to then get comfortable in your own skin to do that.

It's not a vanity thing. It's not a superficial appearance thing, okay? It truly does open up doors for you, and you can improve the quality of your life because you'll become a more open, more vulnerable, more real person that can be seen, and you're not hiding underneath that blanket.

Erin: Well, and I've seen just from you, knowing you since I was nine years old, and then reconnecting with you, to see, "Oh, this is the real Shelley." The weight was in the way. I didn't know the real Shelley. Like I "heard this", and "saw this", and I kept trying to push it all away to get to the real Shelley.

Shelley: Right, Shelley's in there somewhere!

Erin: She's in there. But now that the weight is gone, it's like now *there's* the real Shelley, and I can take her seriously and I can connect with her. Whereas before, I felt that I couldn't do that.

Shelley: The weight was a barrier.

Erin: It was. So, of course I'm thinking, "People obviously can't take me seriously."

Shelley: You then projected that onto yourself saying, "Maybe my weight is also a barrier to other people right now."

Erin: Yeah, because I sensed that people feel uncomfortable around me.

Shelley: Really?

Erin: And I wondered why. You know, the lies we tell ourselves, right? So, "Oh, they're just intimidated by how confident I am."

Well, after engaging you I thought maybe it's that they're trying to say, "The real Erin is in there, but we can't see her." And so, they feel uncomfortable with that. I thought, "Well, I have to prove something to them. They want me to lose weight in order to be legitimate. Well, I'm not gonna do that!"

Shelley: Right. Dang it! That's not polite. That's not politically correct!

Erin: You can't say that to people, you can't do that.

Shelley: "You can't discriminate against me because of my weight!"

Erin: That's right. When the reality is, I'm sensing now...

Shelley: You put up that barrier.

Erin: Well, I have to take ownership of that. I have to take responsibility. Before I could take responsibility for that I had to believe, and then to see, that people really wanted the real Erin.

Shelley: People *do* want the REAL you!

Day 68

"It's day 68 in my weight loss transformation journey with Shelley Johnson, the Losing Coach. And as of today, I've lost 15 pounds!

I missed two weeks of coaching with her, but I felt very confident that I had gotten what I needed. I kept telling her, "I've got this, I can do this." And while I have been diligent in meeting my personal goals and my assignments, those two weeks left me out of the loop of connecting with her and participating with her energy level, her confidence, and her assurance. So, I did myself no favors by doing that.

The one bit of advice I would have is to stay consistent with your coaching because you may think that you can do it on your own, but I just proved to myself that I do need her continual support at this stage.

I need to stay connected to her energy level and clarity because that's what's helping me actualize this potential within me. I'm doing the work, but I need to stay attached to her confidence in being able to keep this moving forward. So, I look forward to another week and check in next week because Shelley continues to engage me with the absolute unwavering confidence of being able to actualize this potential. Thanks, Shelley. I love what you do, and so appreciate who you are!"

Three Months

"This is day 89 in my weight loss transformation journey. I've lost 21 pounds. I've broken through a barrier that, in all of the attempts at losing weight, I've never been able to break before. I broke through 160 pounds! That's a major milestone for me. I knew that if I could break 160 pounds that this was for real. And so here I am. This is for real. Because I've broken 160, I know I'm gonna make it which never before did I think was possible. With Shelley, I know that it's completely possible.

I've clung to her confidence and now I can have it for myself. One of the things that's been so encouraging, and actually very motivating in Shelley's program is that I don't have to bring in a unique set of foods. I eat the same thing everybody else is eating. Just last week, I was at a wedding and I had the champagne, the wedding cake, and the chocolate covered strawberries. And then I went to a cookout and I ate the barbecue and the beans and the baked potatoes, just like everybody else.

In the past, with the other programs I've done, I would go to social functions and have to take my own food and could not eat what everybody else was eating and that made me feel uncomfortable. I felt isolated, I felt set apart, and I felt like attention would be drawn to me. With Shelley's program I look like everybody else, I eat what everybody else is eating, and nobody knows the difference. The only way somebody knows that I'm doing something different is because I look so different.

And I can eat at the same restaurants and participate in the same foods, it's not a separation, I'm not separated, I'm a part of what's going on. So, thank you again, Shelley. To be able to reach this major milestone of breaking through a barrier that I've never been able to break through before on my own, to be able to actually weigh less than what my driver's license says, I know that I'm on my way! I know that this goal is possible, and it's all because of Shelley Johnson and what she's doing in her weight loss program. Thanks, Shelley!"

Five Months

"As of today, I've lost 25 pounds and it feels incredible! It's been exciting to see the progress and *feel* the progress. My body *feels* different and my energy level is different. The way I move in my body is different and the way that I feel about my body is most definitely different. It's exciting to actually feel good about my body, to actually *love* my body, and to be excited about how it looks, and how it's changing.

One of the things I've recently discovered is the power of one-on-one coaching in the weight loss journey. There was a period of time over the summer where I was not able to keep my regular weekly appointments with Shelley and as a result, my progress actually began to slow down. Well, that was wonderful motivation for me to reach out to Shelley and to say, "I really need to be diligent about keeping these appointments." And Shelley said, "Well, I've always been here. So, it's your call."

I explained that I was doing pretty well, but there were a couple of things I wanted to talk to her about.

She said, "No problem. We'll get right to it. Let's go ahead and record your weight."

She said, "How much do you weigh today?"

Though I was actually 155.8 on the scale, I answered her, "I weigh 165.8 pounds." And I felt okay with that.

And she said, "Wow." In her usual non-judgmental style. "What happened?"

I said, "Well, what do you mean, what happened? Isn't that a pound less than last week?"

She said, "Erin, last week you weighed 156.8. that means you've put on nine pounds."

And I said, "Oh, oh Shelley... Now, you want to know how I'm doing? That's what's going on. My brain still does not understand that I'm done with the 160's. That I'll never weigh 160 again. My brain still thinks that I'm in the 160's because I have never broken through the 160's in my adult life."

I told her how much I needed help in being able to reprogram my brain. Right then and there we both understood how vital it was for me to stay connected to her because she was going to keep showing me the progress I was making. She was going to keep pointing out that I am doing it. And when I was stuck, she was going to provide fresh perspectives and creative ideas on how to keep myself motivated and how to actually reprogram my brain to allow me to do the very thing that I longed to do but had never been able to do for myself."

Seven Months

"I love Shelley's plan! It's incredibly simple, it's amazingly doable! What sets it apart is Shelley.

Her ability to stay connected with her clients, and her ability to keep us focused on our goal and to help us stay motivated, and to help us reprogram our brains so we don't sabotage our own efforts. It is absolutely amazing to me. So, Shelley, I'll say it again, I love what you do. Thanks for who you are and thank you for the amazing transformation that you're helping me accomplish. You're helping me make my dreams come true!"

Shelley: It seems like you began just yesterday, but it's Month 7. Seven months, 30 pounds. That has to mean an incredible difference for you and your life. Let's talk about the difference. If you can, take yourself back to when you were almost 180 pounds in March. You came to me. If you can, go back there to that moment of being 180 pounds. Now, you've lost 30 pounds. Seven months later, you've had time to adjust to this. Although, hasn't it flown by?

Erin: It's staggering to me that the time keeps moving. The time is going to keep going, it's going to eventually be December, and then it's gonna be January, because it always does.

Shelley: Time passes. It always does.

Erin: It always comes around.

30 pounds. This is a huge physical difference! 30 pounds is a staggering difference. My toddler weighs 30 pounds, and I pick him up and carry him and think, "I used to carry this around."

And the energy level, it has occurred to me, probably over the last eight weeks, has increased. I'm up at 5:30 in the morning! Just awake.

Shelley: Excited about your day!

Erin: Yeah, yeah!

Shelley: Having lost 30 pounds and being able to move easier and having more energy, those are very specific, tangible results. But now let's talk about this complete metamorphosis you've gone through, because people are saying, "Wow, you've really gone through a metamorphosis!"

Erin: Yeah, the metamorphosis may be shocking to people, but to me it's, I'm finally able to be who I always thought of myself as, who I've always perceived myself to be. This has been me all along, I just couldn't let it out.

Shelley: And let's talk about some of this self-dialogue. I know you have a lot of this self-dialogue in your head. Specifically, again if you can go back to March when you were 180 pounds, I want you to picture yourself standing in front of the mirror. What would be some of that self-dialogue you would have with Erin? You look at her, you see her, what do you say?

Erin: It's just the acknowledgment of, "Well, here we are halfway through life. And you just haven't been able to do it, have you? You just weren't able to do it. I guess you just have to admit that you weren't able to do it."

The other side is frustration. You know, extreme frustration, "*Why* have you not been able to get a handle on this? Why have you not been able to be free of this?" A lot of avoidance. Not knowing what to say, so you just don't say anything. A separateness. There was a lot of separateness. I could not be ...

Shelley: "That's not me, that's not who I want to be. I can't be that."

Erin: Yeah. So, I couldn't be *in* my body. I couldn't be one with my body, I couldn't pay attention to my body.

Shelley: That's what I experienced at 220 pounds. Looking in the mirror and having this kind of denial like, "That's not me. That's not what I want to be. I don't want to be this big, I don't like that. That's not who I am." What a horrible disconnect! What a horrible... Oh, what's the word I'm looking for? When you've got two opposing forces that don't agree with each other? You have a physical... you're seeing in the mirror, and yet on the inside you're screaming, "That's not *me*! That's not who I want to be."

Erin: I call it dissonance. The cognitive dissonance of, "I can't handle that that's me. I have absolutely no idea what to do about that. I have tried everything I know to do." And in so doing, I just wasn't even whole. I was not connected to myself.

Shelley: You cannot be whole if you are not connected with yourself. Being connected with yourself means living according to who you are, what you want, and who you want to be.

And so that cognitive dissonance led to what kind of emotions in you?

Erin: Well, I pretty much shut a lot of the emotions down. I had to say, "I just have to resign myself to the fact that this is irrelevant, even the concept of feeling beautiful. I had decided that beautiful was just irrelevant because I couldn't get myself wrapped around what beautiful was.

Shelley: And look at you now! How do you wrap around that now as beautiful? Like when you look in the mirror now?

Erin: Well, now I'm becoming what I believed myself to be, always who I've wanted to be. And to say, "That is me."

Shelley: Yes, it's YOU!"

~~*~*~*~*~*

And so, Erin got out too.

She was just as afraid as anyone in this escape. She had become very familiar with the prison camp and even found comfort in it. At least she *knew* when the beatings were coming. At least she had the security of knowing what it's like in this prison, where everything was, and what to expect. She was very afraid of yet another failure. She had tried so many times to get out, only to fail, again and again.

I remember in the beginning, she said to me, "I can't risk another failure; I can't emotionally risk it."

I touched her hand and said very quietly, "You won't this time."

She trusted me.

In so doing, she discovered the same path I had discovered, through the same process, and she also escaped. Now I knew my escape wasn't about *me* being *lucky*. It was about this path.

This path was the way out of this prison camp, a path that led to freedom, to a luscious field of green and gold by the riverbank.

The amazing part is I did not direct every step she took or tell her to pick up the pace. I simply stood solid at the end of the path, planted by the riverbank, gently waving her forward, whispering, "It's this way…"

Weight Loss Journey Worksheet

Please be as specific and as descriptive as you can.

1. A word or two that describes how I feel right now:

2. My weight today:

3. What part of yourself did you see in Erin?

4. What can you relate to in Erin's journey?

5. What inspired you most?

6. How did her transformation make you feel?

7. What did she share that gives you hope for yourself?

8. In what ways are you ready to do this for yourself?

9. In what ways are you ready to stop suffering? Haven't you suffered enough?

And if you could use a bit of the non-judgmental, encouraging coaching from Shelley, join Shelley's Club now. She can help. It's this way… www.losingcoach.com

Get Set...

Accept your Appetite is Real

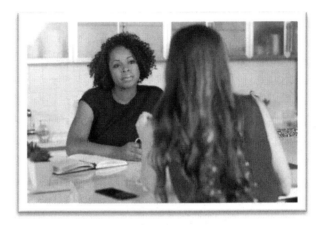

I have so many women tell me they are an emotional and/or stress eater. To which I always reply, "Yeah. So am I. Always have been, still am, and always will be."

I don't even like the phrases "emotional eater" or "stress eater" because it implies there is something psychologically wrong with you.

Like... "*Oh I am such a weak person mentally that I just cannot cope*, so I turn to food."

And that's simply not true. You are not weak and there is

nothing psychologically wrong with you.

An increased appetite for food is controlled by the brain. It's simple science. And it's natural.

You didn't do it. It's not a weakness. It's not a problem.

Read on for some huge relief as you experience a very obvious revelation that you can reduce your own appetite naturally. You will understand that there is nothing wrong with you.

Accept Your Appetite Is Real

Do you think you're a "stress-eater"?

Your body is a scientific machine. When you experience stress or extreme emotion or even fatigue, the body sends a message to the brain saying, "I'm tired, I'm stressed, I'm fatigued." The brain then sends a message to your body to increase your appetite, because it knows that food is a natural antidepressant, it's experienced it before. It knows that food is a natural anti-anxiety solution, it's experienced that before.

When you experience intense emotion, or stress, or fatigue, the brain sends a message to the body "increase your appetite" because *food* is going to make me feel better right now. This is natural, this is science, there is nothing psychologically wrong with you at all by having an increased appetite. *You* didn't do it! Your brain did it! Your brain increased your appetite. It's science!

One time I was extremely stressed and emotional, but interestingly enough, actually had no appetite whatsoever, and didn't eat a thing—when I had the flu! Ha! So, I guess I'm not the "stress-eater" or "emotional eater" I thought I was after all!

Your appetite gets either increased or decreased from the messages from your brain to your body. When you have the flu, your brain sends a message to your body to turn off its appetite to protect you. The brain understands that at that point in time when you have the flu, you're not able to digest anything right now. If you try to eat something you're going to vomit or have diarrhea because you have a stomach bug.

The brain says, "you cannot digest any food right now, so I'm going to turn off your appetite, so you don't eat food." This is controlled by the brain.

An increased appetite or a decreased appetite is a physiological response that we cannot control by sheer willpower. I have had the flu where my stomach's empty and it's growling, but I still have no appetite whatsoever.

Appetite is defined as your desire for food. Plain and simple, your desire for food. So, can you be physically full and have a desire for more food? Yes. Your appetite is very real. That is your desire for more food.

Appetite is your brain's message, your brain's signal of "desire food." Think about that. How many times have you overeaten and stuffed yourself, and you still want more food? Your appetite is very real! *Something* is increasing your appetite, but there is nothing psychologically wrong with you.

The good news is, your brain can decrease your appetite. There are things you can do to train the brain to decrease your appetite... that don't involve getting the flu!

As I learned how to understand and accept my appetite, as something I'm not in control of, I realized it was just like the weather. I could not control my appetite any more than I could control the weather.

On this path out, I couldn't control the weather. Nobody can control the weather, which is why we learn how to be prepared for it, and how to protect ourselves from it.

If I anticipated storms coming, I took shelter. If I had to wait until the storm passed, I was patient. I paid attention to the patterns, bundled up when it got cold, sought higher ground when it rained, and stayed low during high winds.

I was learning how to be prepared and protect myself. I was getting set.

Accept your Appetite is Real Worksheet

1. A word or two that describes how I feel right now.

2. My weight today:

3. Do you see that there is nothing psychologically wrong with you?

4. What is the definition of appetite?

5. What controls your appetite?

6. What physical feelings do you experience that send a message to your brain to increase your appetite?

7. What emotional feelings do you experience that send a message to your brain to increase your appetite?

8. Why does the brain increase the appetite as a result of these feelings?

9. Do you accept that you are not at fault for your appetite?

Remember, if you want personal, inspirational, non-judgmental support from Shelley, join Shelley's Club now. She can help. It's this way... www.losingcoach.com

Articulate Your Higher Purpose

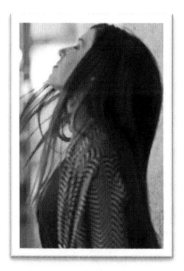

This is not a religious program, so you don't need to
believe in God to do it.

I am simply sharing the next thing I did in my own
process...along with shutting out the diet industry
advice, deciding to keep it private, and realizing there
was nothing psychologically wrong with me, I wrote a letter to
God.

This is your next step. Write a letter to God, the Universe, yourself...whatever/whoever you want. I've had clients write it to God, their "best self", their guardian angel, and even a deceased parent.

I call it "Letter to God" because I wrote my letter to God (my divine source of unconditional LOVE). Please write this letter to *whoever* you feel comfortable writing it to. I am not here to tell you who or what to believe in spiritually. This *will* be a spiritual experience for you, but the specifics of it are up to you.

Keep reading to understand what this Letter to God is and what you should include in it.

Shelley's Letter to God

I have to back up here and tell you a little bit about my story, then this is going to be your assignment this week. So, rewind to January 2006. I'm 220 pounds, and I was miserable and depressed. Quite honestly, I had been hit with many arrows in life. Not trying to have a pity party, but life was difficult, and life was stressful, and life was overwhelming me. I was under a lot of judgement.

One, I had experienced quite a bit of medical trauma. I had experienced judgement and self-condemnation—there was a tremendous amount of guilt that I was carrying around over the birth of my child and not being a good enough mother. Two, I had been mistreated by people.

I was observing all of that thinking it was my fault, thinking that I was bringing it on myself, and thinking it all sucked! Life sucked, and there was a lot of guilt attached to that. There was so much self-judgement. And again, a lot of arrows, actually arrows inflicted by other people. But because these arrows were things I believed about myself, that I deserved it and I wasn't a good enough mother, and I was not good enough in any way, I believed that this was just the way I was meant to be treated.

With the accumulation of all that judgement, I was in a very miserable, miserable place. And despite the outside sources of it, I knew down deep that my misery was because of my weight. My weight was the core of my misery.

I was aware and said to myself, "Look, I have a lot of problems I can't solve right now, and I know if I lose weight, I *still* can't solve all my problems. I know losing weight doesn't solve all your problems. I know that!"

But intuitively, I knew if I could lose weight, I could at least *deal with* them. I'd have the confidence and strength to *cope with* my problems. But I couldn't do any coping with where I was. I couldn't lose weight and I couldn't cope. And the worst part, I also knew I couldn't be thin tomorrow.

So here I am, 220 pounds, miserable. I think it was the night, too, that I couldn't breathe. It was the night I'd eaten too much, and my jeans were cutting off my circulation, and I couldn't breathe. God, at that point, I'm like, "What the heck? I'm physically miserable. I am emotionally depleted, and in all ways depleted—mentally, spiritually, emotionally, physically. I am just as low as I can be. I'm completely miserable. I'm so depressed!"

Well, what's natural to think when you're in a place like that? I want to check out. It's too much. Life's too hard at this point.

It wasn't that I didn't love people, life had just been too hard on me. I couldn't handle it. I was done, and I wanted to check out right then and there, but I didn't know how or what I was going to do. It's just the way I felt.

I realized the heart and the head don't always agree. My heart was feeling so much pain, screaming, "I want out!"

My head was saying very calmly, "You can't do that. You have children."

"I know I have children, and I love them so much. Still, this is so painful for me, this life! I'm fat! So-and-so's mistreating me... 'This' is going on. And 'this' situation's not going to get resolved any time soon. I mean, I can't get out of this situation! It seems like everyone hates me."

That's pretty much how I felt, like everyone hated me. My son has a disability and it's all my fault. How am I ever going to change that? I can't reverse this. His life is now more difficult because of me. I don't know if I can ever live with myself. I mean, literally, it was a point of—I can't live with myself right now.

I broke down. I started crying. I resolved, "Okay, if I can't kill myself, then I obviously need another option!"

I heard myself say in my head, "God, I need another option!"

But I didn't know what it was. I just knew I needed one.

So, I hit my knees.

I prayed. I grew up in church. I know how to pray. But at that moment in time, I had no words for what I was feeling. It was so enormous.

But I hit my knees. I remember, I was still crying. I mean, I was sobbing crying! I bowed my head, and then I looked up. I kind of remember doing this type of thing, looking up and looking down. I'm looking up because I need help, but I'm bowing my head out of humility and surrender.

I uttered the only three words I could, "God help me."

Because literally at that moment, I was about to make a decision that I knew I'd regret, and I needed another option.

GOD HELP ME!

Now remember, logically, I was saying, "I know I can't do this", but it's still how my heart felt.

So that was it. I prayed, "God help me!"

I don't know if God answered my prayer right then and there. Do I believe He did? Yeah, because I was in a pretty humble place, a place of true humility, a place of, "Okay, I'm surrendered, face down on the ground. What else do you want me to do?"

But anyway, I got up off my knees, and I grabbed a notebook, just a simple spiral-bound notebook. And I wrote God a letter.

In this letter, everything, and I mean everything, just poured out. Every emotion that I felt, everything that I wanted, everything that I experienced, I was letting God know. He already knew anyway. It wasn't like I could hide this from Him, but I expressed it. I wrote it all out, every detail, every raw, emotional feeling, I wrote it all out, probably for the first time.

In all these nights that I prayed, "God, help me lose weight," I thought I was expressing it, but it was only a trite prayer. Now was the first time that I was really truthful in *expressing* it emotionally, honestly and completely unfiltered.

I talked about the pain. I talked about my past. I talked about my experiences— "I never play outside with my kids. I'm embarrassed. I'm ashamed. I'm mad. I can't do anything anymore. My back hurts. I don't even go to church anymore because I have no clothes to wear. This is a stumbling block to me, God."

It wasn't that I was rude or angry at God, I was honest in how I felt, because I figured, "What was wrong with my feelings anyways?" They were my feelings.

This letter was my turning point. It was my point of true surrender. It was cathartic. And it opened the door to all of my success.

In this letter to God I want you to write this week, I want you to talk about the past and how being overweight has hurt you, because you wouldn't be here if it hadn't hurt you. You wouldn't be here if it hasn't caused you suffering.

In my letter to God, I talked about the past, I talked about the present, and I talked about the future.

1. Past
2. Present
3. Future

I talked about what I wanted and why I wanted it.

What do you want and why do you want it?

"Well, I want to be healthy. I want to be happy. I want to play with my kids. I want to feel good about myself. I want to be confident."

Me being overweight caused a lot of suffering, and I expressed that to God. Again, He already knows. You're not hiding anything by not letting Him know. Again, past, present, and future.

And—What do you want and why do you want it? Make your requests known.

Here are some helpful parameters for your assignment:

There's no length requirement, but it should be substantial, maybe around four to six pages, give or take, in your notebook.

The point is to be *real, raw, and honest.*

The more emotion you express, the better. We're not going to stay here; we're not going to ruminate in this past.

I also want you to be sure to include these three elements somewhere in your letter:

1. Express gratitude

2. Ask for help
3. Promise something in exchange, for example, to give credit to your higher power

These three elements in your letter are *very important* and can be included anywhere in your letter.

Please don't put this assignment off and please don't rush through it. I encourage you to set aside a substantial amount of time to write this letter.

I didn't know it at the time, but my letter was kind of like a message in a bottle.

On this path, I was like a pioneer embarking on un-tread territory. I wrote the letter to ask for help, to document where I was at the moment. I sent it off to sea, with the intention of only God finding it. God *is* the only one who found it. Nobody has ever read my personal letter to God. It is still just only between me and God.

Get set... write your letter and articulate your higher purpose now.

Articulate Your Higher Purpose Worksheet

Please be specific and as descriptive as you can.

Answer these questions about what you are thinking and feeling and include them in your letter. Write your "Letter to God" in a notebook or journal or separate word document. The length is to be substantial. The more real, raw, and emotional, the better. Take your time but complete it as soon as you can.

1. A word or two that describes how I feel right now:

2. My weight today:

3. How has being overweight affected your life?

4. How have you suffered in the past?

5. What are you feeling right now in the present?

6. What do you want in the future and why do you want it?

7. Express gratitude.

8. Ask for help.

9. Give credit where credit is due. Promise to give the credit to your higher power.

It's ok to reach out for help. If you need personal support from Shelley to continue down this path, join Shelley's Club now. She can help. It's this way… www.losingcoach.com

GO!

The Process from A to Z

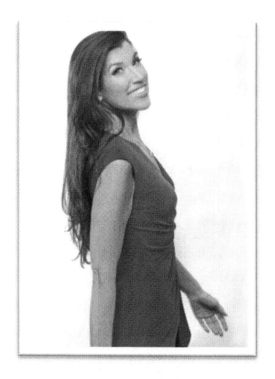

H ave you experienced a decreased appetite yet?

We've removed some of your anxiety around weight loss by equipping you to not listen to the diet industry.

We've protected you by giving you permission to respect your privacy.

Inspired you through Erin's weight loss journey.

Validated your experiences with your appetite.

And given you a very key assignment in writing your Letter to God.

Perhaps you are seeing weight loss success already. If not, have no fear. Tomorrow will be the day you do, and now we are going to prepare you for it.

The worksheet for this chapter has very important instructions for tomorrow, or for when you do go on to the next chapter.

Take these instructions seriously. I'm so excited for what you are about to experience! I want to be with you in spirit...you are about to cross a very significant threshold.

The Process from A to Z

If you're here to find out how to lose weight, I'm going to tell you right here and now. Not only can I tell you in one sentence, I can tell you in two words—EAT LESS.

Yes, that's right! Eat less. You already know this. That's not why you're here, to hear that. Everyone knows this. And in case you don't believe me, I could lock you up in a cage on a deserted island and prove that eating less will result in weight loss to you really quickly!

See, you don't need someone to tell you *how* to lose weight, because you know how. You're not wanting to know "how to" lose weight. What you're wanting is the *how to the how to… how* do you eat less on a day-in and day-out basis over time to result in the weight loss you desire?

This is what you want. You simply want the *ability* to eat less. You've been convinced you must go *do* something to lose weight. But you discover very quickly, nothing you can do will give you weight loss results if you're eating more.

You want the ability to eat less. And the good news is, eating less can actually be pretty effortless if your appetite is decreased. (You know like when you have the stomach flu, and your brain turns off your appetite for a while, it's super easy to eat less.)

How do you do that?

You train the brain. You simply train the brain. That's my entire process.

It's funny, people would ask me, "How did you lose weight?"

And I'm like, "I can't answer that question. How am I supposed to answer that question? Do you want me to tell you scientifically? Emotionally? Psychologically? Spiritually? I can't answer that question. It was so many things."

The ability to eat less came from everything I was doing.

So now you're saying, "I need the ability to do this for myself. I need the ability to put this into practice". This is a process that will give you this ability and train your brain to decrease your appetite.

It's a process. There is no pat answer. I really cannot tell you how I lost weight until you go through the process. And you experience it. Because it's going to train your brain. The process itself trains your brain, which will decrease your appetite, which will give you the ability to put into practice the very thing that you long to do, which is to eat less, to lose weight.

That's what you want to do. It's so simple. The science is simple. The psychological part of it. The emotional part of it. The spiritual part of it. All parts of it are really very simple. But it's not just one thing.

Again, if it was one thing, if it was just science, then I could send you to my deserted island, and you could lose weight there. Or I could lock you to a hospital bed and not feed you. I mean, either way, that's the science. Eat less. That's no big secret. You know that.

But how do you do that? How do you do that, day in and day out, to give yourself the results that you want? Because you know intuitively, "look, this comes down to the decisions that I make every day." Doesn't it?

The brain follows patterns. People say habits, I just don't like that word because it sounds a little judgmental. The brain follows the path of least resistance. In order to *train* it to have new habits, in order to train it to follow a new pathway, you have to walk down that pathway a number of times, again and again and again. And then THAT pathway becomes the path of least resistance for your brain to follow.

That is really the difference with this process. I'm telling you, you don't have to put your life on hold for it. You don't have to go do something different. You don't have to buy special food. You don't have to drink shakes, take supplements, or do anything crazy. Literally, you can do this on your own!

You just implement the steps. You put the process into practice, and it's not hard. It's simple.

It's *not* hard. You put the process into practice, you're going to see the results right away, and it's going to encourage you, you're going to feel good about it, it's a happy program! It's a very, very happy program!

You'll be able to take this and fit it into your lifestyle. You can't try to fit your lifestyle into a diet, rather you must fit your diet into your lifestyle. You're going to create your own diet! And that makes it sound more difficult than it is. It's really not!

Now this will sound like I'm speaking out of both sides of my mouth, and I am! It's simple and easy! It really is... *and* it requires time, commitment, effort, and thinking!

Yes, it's going to require you thinking!

It's going to require using your brain! Everyone has a brain they can use! You have memories, ideas, information. And it really is about making informed decisions. It really is about making the decisions that you want to make on a day-in and day-out basis for yourself.

Because that's where you feel the frustration—I didn't do what I wanted to do! I wanted to make *this* decision, and then I ended up doing something else. And it wasn't in keeping with the decision I *wanted* to make. Which, the decision you want to make is to eat less so you can lose weight. And then you end up not doing it, and when you end up not doing it, you go "Oh! Why'd I do that?"

It's about making informed decisions with LOVE. This is how I explain it to a client.

~~*~*~*~*~*

Shelley: You do that every day for your baby. You make all kinds of informed decisions with LOVE for her. And how well are you taking care of her?

Client: Pretty good!

Shelley: Oh, pretty good? You only ensure her survival and her health!

So, it's going to be the same thing! You have everything you need right now. There's nothing you need outside of yourself to lose weight. There's no product, no shake, no workout regimen. Everything you need to lose weight is inside of you right now at this very minute. It's deep inside of you.

And what we're going to do is raise it up from your core to the front of your mind. And we're going to put it at this level of your awareness, (pointing to forehead) in the front of your mind.

You're going to have a conscious awareness of the decisions you're going to make. And it's going to make all the difference. Again, informed decisions with LOVE.

It's like the yin and the yang, the law and the grace, the faith and the works, one is dead without the other. You need the entire process. Because again, you could put the science into practice, but without the grace, how do you continue if the science isn't perfect?

And I know you're here right now thinking you've made a lot of bad decisions. So, we're going to remove the judgement off of you. That's the first thing that we do. The removal of judgement —you're going to discover how huge that is!

I hear ads on the radio spouting, "Come join our gym, it's a judgement-free zone."

And I'm like, "No... you have no idea."

See, if I'm a 200 lb. woman and I go to your gym, trust me, I'm going to feel judged. It's uncomfortable, intimidating, and who wants to experience that?

This is a safe program. It's comfortable. I'm here to protect you and make this safe. In secret. Because, just like in the womb, your new life will be woven together in secret.

And I'm going to equip you with the tools.

You will be walking this path on your own, but I'm going to be there. Because I've been there. I've walked this path. I've lost the weight. And I've helped many women lose their own weight.

I know what it is to walk this path. I'm going to be there to say, "It's this way..."

I know exactly where you are. Exactly what you're feeling. All the frustration, all the pain, all the despair. All the self-judgement that you're feeling right now. I know the tears that you cry at night when you go to bed. I know the self-condemnation. We're our own worst critic. And I know what you say to yourself.

And people that haven't been there… the people who have never experienced that, they don't know the pain that a woman feels in her heart when it comes to her body being overweight, and how shameful that feels to us. And yet, we have to walk out into the world, and the world gets to see it. And we walk around with this cloud of shame, that we've let ourselves go.

No one talks about that. What they talk about is: just accept yourself the way you are, you're beautiful, embrace your curves. And I can try to do that all day long, and yet, I'm still ashamed of my body.

And people that don't know that, that haven't experienced that… they don't know what it's like. It's like trying to get from A to Z. And they can tell you all day long what it's like to be at Z. When you hire your personal trainer, or your nutritionist, they can tell you all day long, "Well this is how you eat at Z, this is how you work out at Z." And they have no idea what it's like to be at A. And you're going, "Great, if I could get there, I would. But I'm not there yet."

So, I train you to go from A to Z, because I've been at A. And I don't even talk about Z. I don't tell you what to eat. I don't tell you how to work out. That's up to you. I respect you. I respect your own decisions that you make.

That's kinda new, too. Respecting your decisions. Because if someone's telling you to follow a diet, eat this, do that, they're not respecting the decisions that your brain is fully capable of making for yourself.

Because listen, they don't live where you live. They don't have the same friends, and same events, and social outings, and job and husband that you have. They don't know what you go through. So how can they tell you what to do?

This is really about your weight loss independence and making your own decisions. In your life. With your family. In your situation.

~~*~*~*~*

At the beginning of this path, I was at A, right after I crawled underneath the fence. I could not see the end of the path. I couldn't think about it, talk about it, or even worry about it. I focused on exactly where I was and taking one step at a time.

I knew the journey would take time, and it wouldn't happen overnight. I embraced it, step by step, stone by stone; and I rested when I needed to. I knew I'd reach the end of the path if I just kept going. And I did. You will too. Embrace the journey and the path you're on.

It's GO time!

It's this way...

The Process from A to Z - Instructions for Tomorrow

Check off that you have read and understood all of your instructions for the next chapter.

1. One or two words to describe how I feel right now:

2. My weight today:

3. Please read the next chapter on a special day around noon or sometime between 11 a.m. - 2 p.m.

4. Tonight, or tomorrow morning, take a "Before" photo.

5. Please weigh yourself at home first thing in the morning and write down your weight in your notebook.

6. Please fast for 8-12 hours before you experience the next chapter. If you read the next chapter at Noon tomorrow, do not eat after midnight tonight. Coffee, Water, Tea are okay (No sugar or cream). If you need to take medication that is to be taken with food, do as your doctor/prescription instructs. If you start to feel light-headed, grab something to eat. Otherwise, please fast for half a day so you are skipping one meal right before you read the next chapter. Understand this is a one-time thing and you will never be asked to do this again. Understand that you can and will eat shortly after you experience the next chapter.

7. What thoughts do you have right now?

You don't have to go it alone. If you want personal, inspirational, non-judgmental coaching from Shelley, join Shelley's Club now. She can help. It's this way... www.losingcoach.com

Steps 1, 2, & 3...

Power, Truth and Love

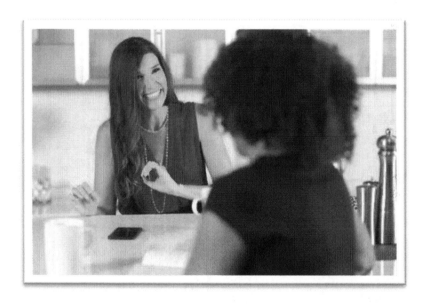

T he HOW, WHAT, and WHY to weight loss mastery are revealed in the first three steps of the Losing Coach process.

You will learn:

The POWER to lose weight. It's already inside you!

The TRUTH is *what* you need to focus on. It's not what you think!

And LOVE is *why* you will be able to do it. This is what makes the Losing Coach process *different* from anything else you've used to lose weight!

Let Power, Truth and LOVE change the way you think about weight loss forever.

The Truth About Weight Loss
Power, Truth and Love

I'm not a trainer and I'm not a nutritionist. I teach women the process that I created to lose 90 pounds all on my own, without a diet, without a product, without a trainer and no gimmicks. The mission of Losing Coach is to help women lose weight. I do that by teaching them the truth about weight loss.

I used to weigh 220 pounds. I know what it's like to be overweight, and all the emotional and physical pain that goes along with it. Overweight from childhood, I longed to be thin and feel beautiful. I spent over 30 years of my life wishing I could change.

After a series of unfortunate events, including a rare disease during pregnancy, giving birth to premature babies, a near death experience, and a hysterectomy at 34 years of age, I lost myself inside a body I was trapped in. I was in pain, emotionally, spiritually, and physically.

But in 2006 without a trainer, without a nutritionist, without following a diet, without gimmicks, I lost 90 pounds on my own.

How did I do it? I coached myself. I taught myself how to remove the mental and emotional blocks that were preventing me from permanently losing weight.

I've maintained that 90-pound loss ever since. I not only lost weight in a healthy way but was able to do it permanently. While so doing, I developed a process that will help any woman do the same.

My mission is to show women from all walks of life, no matter what you've tried in the past, no matter what you've been through, no matter how many times you failed before, no matter how much you weigh, you can lose weight simply and without products or gimmicks or dieting. You can lose weight on your own and keep it off for good by learning the truth about weight loss.

What you are about to read is an actual Losing Coach workshop with real women just like you. I take them through the first steps I took to remove the mental and emotional blocks that kept me from losing weight.

Step 1 – POWER

Delay for a Greater Purpose

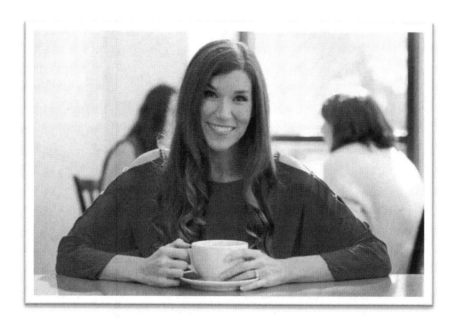

In this Losing Coach workshop session, I will show how your brain makes decisions and why you take action. This process occurs every day of your life.

Workshop participants are instructed to stop eating after midnight the night before the workshop and to bring a snack with them to eat during the workshop. It's a one-time event and they never have to do it again.

I show them how following that simple instruction unlocks their personal ability to lose weight and how they can access that ability anytime they want. I begin by asking the participants how they feel.

~~*~*~*~*~*

Shelley: How do you feel? I mean emotionally, physically, anything.

Participant: Fat.

Participant: Tired.

Participant: Chubby.

Participant: Pathetic.

Shelley: Mm-hmm (affirmative). Pathetic?

Participant: Hungry.

Participant: Good one.

Shelley: *Hungry*? Why do you feel hungry?

Participant: You asked us not to eat anything.

Shelley: (Bewildered) You didn't eat anything today?

Participant: No.

Shelley: (pointing at another participant) Did you?

Participant: No. I did have a bite of a little banana without even thinking about it. I was cutting it up for my daughter and thought, oh, I wasn't supposed to eat anything.

Shelley: Then you stopped?

Participant: I did, I did. I was like, "Okay, can't eat that one." My daughter had the rest of them.

Shelley: (To another participant) You ate nothing?

Participant: Nothing.

Shelley: What about you?

Participants: Water. I had black coffee. Water.

Shelley: You didn't eat anything today?

Participant: No.

Shelley: Do you know what time it is?

Participant: Yes.

Shelley: You feel hungry?

Participant: Mm-hmm (Very affirmative).

Shelley: But you didn't eat anything?

Participant: Right.

Shelley: Anyone else hungry?

Participants: Yes!

Shelley: Why didn't you eat anything?

Participant: I was told not to. Same reason.

Shelley: Okay. *Wow!* Why did you listen to me?

Participant: I figured if I ate it was going to ruin the bloodwork.

Shelley: If I tried to take your blood, it would be really, really bad! (laughter)

I'm not trained to be a nurse or a doctor. I've never had any of that training whatsoever. It would be painful for both of us! Let's see here. Let's talk about this reason...

You mentioned *reason*. You trusted me. Isn't it the same as when your doctor tells you not to eat before a test or procedure? What is your core belief about that?

Participant: Some good is going to come out of it.

Participant: There's a purpose for it.

Shelley: Ah, you just gave me chills, did you see that?

That's the first key word: **Purpose**. Okay?

This was your core *belief* about the instruction. That there was a greater *purpose* to not eating this morning. And you made this decision not to eat this morning.

You made this decision not to eat all on your own! I didn't slap anyone's hand. I wasn't with you this morning. I didn't sew anyone's mouth shut. I gave you an instruction, you believed there was a greater purpose to it, and you did it!

So, you had the core belief there was a greater **purpose**.

We're going to get to nine keywords here when we're done. We're going to have rows of our *key* words, our *decision* words, and in the third row, these words all start with the letter E, to represent how and why you made this decision with such *ease*.

<u>Key:</u>

<u>Decision:</u>

<u>Ease:</u>

Each of you made the decision not to eat this morning with relative ease. When I asked how you were feeling, no one gave me the word "distressed", or "anxious". Was it fun being hungry? Probably not. Do you *feel* hungry? Yes, but that's okay. You accepted that and each of you made the decision to not eat this morning with *ease*. The 'E' word associated with purpose is **"embrace"**.

You *embraced* your core belief that there was a greater purpose to this instruction/decision you made.

Let me point something out to you. All of you so embraced your core belief that there was a greater purpose to this instruction that not a one of you asked me "why"! "Why are you asking me not to eat, Shelley?" *Nobody* asked me that! Even when I'm begging each of you for a reply to my email, *nobody* asked me why!

Participant reacts with embarrassment.

Shelley: I love your reaction! You're thinking, "You're right, I didn't! I didn't ask why!"

It's alright, don't feel stupid, everyone feels the same way. Nobody ever asks me why. And it's okay. Understand you didn't ask why because when you embrace your **belief** in a greater purpose, there is no reason to ask why!

Key: **Purpose**

Decision: **Belief**

Ease: **Embrace**

This exercise we are beginning is a decision-making analysis exercise. I'm breaking down the decision that your brain made in a split second to not eat. You probably made this decision multiple times this morning. I'm showing you how you made this decision. You don't realize it's because the pathways in the brain work pretty fast.

Shelley (To participant/neurologist): You're a neurologist… right? They work fast?

Neurologist: Yes!

Shelley: You're not aware of the brain process in the decision you made this morning, and I'm breaking it down for you.

Shelley (To participant who had banana): You made a decision to put that piece of banana down. And I'll show you how. Because there is something you knew about the instruction. Something I told you. What did you *know* about the instruction?

Now you can only know facts. I'm no longer talking about what you believe in. What did you *know*?
What was some of the self-dialogue you had with yourself in making the decision not to eat? You're a great example because you actually had to put something down. Do you know what you said to yourself?

Participant: That we're going to have a snack later. Oh yeah. I can deal with that.

Shelley: Gave me chills again. What does that mean?

Participant: That we were eventually going to eat.

Shelley: Yes, which means the instruction is... what? That you're going to eat later, that it's what? Not going to last forever?

Participant: Right, right, right. It's temporary.

Shelley: Yeah, there we go, temporary! **Temporary.** This was the *knowledge* that you had about it. I told you in the email. I said this is a one-time thing, and I'm never going to ask you to do this again. You can bring a snack, you can eat later, I promise.

You had the knowledge it was *temporary*.

That's what you said to yourself when you set down the banana!

Participant: Yeah.

Shelley: That's what **empowered** you to do it. You were empowered not to eat this morning because you knew it was temporary. Again, there was no anxiety, no distress. My goodness, if I was told I could never eat again, I would be freaking out! I would be very distressed and anxious, because to never eat again means I die of starvation! You had the *knowledge* that it was *temporary* and that's how you were empowered to follow the instruction and *make this decision* to not eat.

Key:	Purpose	**Temporary**
Decision:	Belief	**Knowledge**
Ease:	Embrace	**Empowered**

~~*~*~*~*~*

Erin: What do you think so far? So simple and obvious. I know. That's how I felt when Shelley began to coach me. Everything she said was so obvious, so simple and yet, so powerful for me. You're beginning to discover how to lose weight now. You are beginning to discover that the power to do it has been inside you all along.

Shelley is going to continue helping us understand this. She asks the participants to remember the times they've been tired. Do the same right now, think about a time you've been tired. That's easy, isn't it? Watch how Shelley uses our familiarity with the feeling of being tired and applies it to weight loss.

~~*~*~*~*~*

Shelley: Has anyone here ever felt tired before?

Participants: All the time! Yes!

Shelley: Even in the afternoon?

Participants: Yes!

Shelley: You feel tired in the afternoon... but you don't take a nap?

Participant: Right. Typically.

Shelley: Because you're working?

Participant: I'm working, right.

Shelley: Do you believe there's a greater purpose in working?
Participant: Yes.

Shelley: Do you know that feeling tired is temporary?

Participant: Yes.

Shelley: Okay. (To another participant) You have a small baby, a girl, right?

Participant: Yes.

Shelley: Okay. Do you ever have to get up with her in the middle the night?

Participant: Yes.

Shelley: Okay, do you ever have to get up at like three a.m. because she is hungry or something?

Participant 2: Yep.

Shelley: Does that make you feel tired?

Participant 2: Yep. That's why I try to see if she can cry it out a little bit. Turn down the monitor a little bit... but then, "okay... she needs me!"

Shelley: You've gotten up in the middle the night even when you're tired?

Participant 2: Yes.

Shelley: You don't just ignore her?

Participant 2: No.

Shelley: So, you just *accept* it? Feeling tired? You just *accept* feeling tired at three a.m.? Or in the middle of the afternoon?

Participant 2: Yeah.

Shelley, to another participant: And you've been tired before?

Participant 3: Yep!

Shelley: And you just accept it?

Participant 3: Part of life.

Shelley: Part of life, right?

The third keyword is **Feeling**.

Do you know what a feeling is? I want you to think about feeling tired. A feeling is an indicator, a *message*, a valid message from the body to the brain, that says, in the case of feeling tired, "I haven't gotten enough sleep." You *feel tired...* so you make the decision to go get me some more sleep!

But you know when you're feeling tired, it's temporary, and eventually you'll catch up on your sleep. You accept it.

That's how you're able to take care of a baby at three a.m., go to work all day, commit to school and work with anything and everything that you do that makes you feel tired. You know it's temporary, so you accept it. Because literally, if it wasn't temporary, if you didn't catch up on your sleep, truth is, you could die of sleep deprivation.

I keep looking at the neurologist... *Right?*

Neurologist: Right!

Shelley: *Feeling hungry* is also a feeling, just like feeling tired. If you feel hungry right now, your body's communicating to your brain, "I have not eaten enough food today." It's a *message*. And it's a valid indicator. It's completely valid!

Just as much as feeling tired is because you haven't gotten enough sleep or you're working too hard and you don't have enough rest, feeling hungry is the same thing. It's a valid, valid feeling. It's a **reaction**!

It's a **reaction** to your **experience**. The Decision word is **Reaction**. The Ease word is **Experience**.

Key:	Purpose	Temporary	**Feeling**
Decision:	Belief	Knowledge	**Reaction**
Ease:	Embrace	Empowered	**Experience**

If you punch me in the stomach and I *experience* being punched in the stomach, I'm going to have the *reaction* of *feeling* pain. If I don't get enough sleep and I have that experience, I'm going to have the reaction of feeling tired. So, if you *experience* not eating, you will have the *reaction* of *feeling* hungry.

But you all *accept* when you feel tired. Why? Because I get the paycheck I'm working for. I've got a child I'm taking care of. I've got a greater purpose going on, so I'm willing to accept when I feel tired and make the decision to keep working or get up in the middle of the night. We do this, make decisions like this, every day of our lives.

Let's talk a little more about this keyword—**Feeling**. Let me ask you, are feelings voluntary or involuntary?

Participant 1: Uhhh...

Participant 2: Voluntary!

Participant 3: Involuntary!

Participant 4: Both?

Shelley: Feelings are 100% *involuntary*. Now I need a volunteer.

Volunteer: Okay, I'll volunteer!

Shelley: Thank you! Alright, role-play with me here, if you will. Let's say I come over to you and I *punch* you in the stomach right now! What are you going to feel?

Volunteer: Pain.

Shelley: Pain. Is that pain voluntary or involuntary?

Volunteer: Involuntary!

Shelley: Right. Now what are you going to do?

Volunteer: I don't know.

Shelley: No seriously, what are you going to do? Punch me back? Or run away?

Volunteer: Probably run away.

Shelley: Right. Because I just punched you and caused you pain, I'm now a threat to you. I doubt you will just stand there and accept that. Are you going to accept that?

Volunteer: No!

Shelley: So, you have one of two choices to make. You either fight back or run and get the heck out of here. You're now in fight or flight. What is fight or flight?

Volunteer: Stress.

Shelley: Right. Now you are experiencing stress. You must fight or take flight. That creates *anxiety*.

But *now*… let's pretend I say to you, "Okay, listen, if you let me punch you in the stomach again, yes, you'll experience pain. But really, I'm not that strong, so it's not going to kill you, you'll survive, and if you let me punch you in the stomach, I'm going to pay you *10 million dollars*!!" Now what are you going to do?

Volunteer: (laughing) Well I'd say, "Bring it on!!"

Shelley: Oh… so *now* you're going to *accept* feeling pain, because you know it's temporary, and there might be a greater purpose in 10 million dollars for you?

Volunteer: Yes!

Shelley: So now, you make this decision to agree to being punched in the stomach while experiencing pain, which is certainly no fun, and *painful*. But now you accept it with *no anxiety*! You will accept the punch without fighting back or running away, without fight or flight, you say "Bring it on!" Complete acceptance. Correct?

Volunteer: Yep!

Shelley: Perfect! *This* **ladies, is exactly how you can make decisions for yourself for weight loss. We're going to eliminate anxiety. Anxiety is what increases your appetite.**

So, we're going to *accept* **our feelings, whether we enjoy them or not, to get rid of the fight or flight, the anxiety, and make decisions with ease.**

I just asked if everyone here has felt tired before, right? That's your involuntary reaction to an experience of working too hard or not getting enough sleep. Hunger is also an involuntary reaction.

Now what you do with that feeling, that involuntary reaction…. whether you *accept* it or not will determine your level of anxiety. Again, anxiety increases your appetite. That's what this process will decrease.

Anxiety is what you've experienced with other diet programs, and why you find your appetite increased while you have tried to diet. You're trying to make "good choices", but you "fight" your involuntary reactions. There is little or no acceptance, so you find yourself in fight or flight, or anxiety, which increases your appetite. And you even judge yourself for these involuntary reactions, "I shouldn't feel hungry", or "I shouldn't feel angry" and all of that judgement continues to increase your appetite.

So, what we will be doing in this process is learning to accept our involuntary reactions, our feelings. This applies to both physical and emotional feelings. They are all involuntary reactions, whether physical or emotional. If you feel angry because someone is rude to you, it's an involuntary reaction. If you feel sad, hurt, disappointed, all involuntary reactions to your experiences. We will learn how to accept them all. This will decrease your anxiety, which will then decrease your appetite.

Accepting (or not accepting) our reactions is just one part of this decision-making process. Our feelings are merely the involuntary, valid indicators. But what decision we ultimately make is based on what we believe, what we know, and how we react to our experiences.

We make all of our decisions in life based on what we *believe*, what we *know*, and how we *react*. These are our **DECISION** words—**belief, knowledge,** and **reaction**.

You all made the decision not to eat this morning. You think you were just following my instruction. But I wasn't with you this morning. I didn't slap your hand when you had the banana in it.

You made the decision to put it down, to not eat it.

You did this on your own. You made this decision all by yourself. This is what your brain did in a split second. All I'm doing is bringing to light some self-dialogue you had with yourself. You've been doing this your whole life, for all the things that had a greater purpose for you.

And this is how this is all going to come together, in one sentence:

You made the **decision** to not eat this morning with **ease** because you **embraced** your core **belief** there was a greater **purpose** and you were **empowered** to *accept* your **reaction** of **feeling** hungry to your **experience** of not eating because you had the **knowledge** it was **temporary**.

So now connect these words in BOLD in the diagram with a continuous curve:

Because you **EMBRACED** your core **BELIEF** in a greater **PURPOSE**, and had the **KNOWLEDGE** your **EXPERIENCE** of not eating, while accepting your involuntary **REACTION** of **FEELING** hungry, was **TEMPORARY**, you were **EMPOWERED** to make this decision to delay your eating, which you EMBRACED.

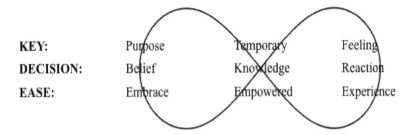

KEY:	Purpose	Temporary	Feeling
DECISION:	Belief	Knowledge	Reaction
EASE:	Embrace	Empowered	Experience

Do you see what symbol we have there? It's the infinity symbol. This is the power of the infinite inside of you, the higher power inside of you that empowers you to make these decisions for yourself, based on what you believe, what you know, and how you react. This is the infinite power of God inside of you.

This is the **HOW**. *How* you are going to lose weight? Right there.

By using the infinite power inside of you to make the decisions you want to make that bring about the desires of your heart.

And it's never going to be this difficult again.

This process is about *delay*, never deprivation.

It's only going to be about delay, like you did today. Literally, let me play this out for you. It's going to be, "Hmm, I feel a little hungry, it's three o'clock in the afternoon, I know I'm eating dinner at five, okay. I can accept this and delay my eating."

This is STEP 1. **POWER** - the *How*.

Do you realize that anything you've ever succeeded at, anything you've ever accomplished, has come from this? It's from the infinite power inside of you to make decisions, and the accumulation of these decisions over time, that bring about the outcome you desire.

If you've earned a degree, succeeded in a career, raised children, or achieved any kind of personal success in your life, it has come from all the decisions you accumulated over time—to stay up late studying, to work over-time, to get up in the middle of the night to take care of children. You've done this already. You just didn't know you could apply this *power* to weight loss.

I hate to sound cheesy, but... you've had the power all along, Dorothy!

Erin: Delay, not deprivation. The power has been inside me all along. When Shelley gave me this decision-making analysis, it was a lightbulb moment for me. I discovered that it wasn't self-control I was lacking, it wasn't more discipline I needed, it was just an understanding that I could accept my reaction to what I was feeling based on what I believe and know. And I did it every day, all day long, in every other area of my life. It's how I got through school. It's how I keep a job, and it's how I fulfill all of my responsibilities and obligations.

I had the ability to do these things, I just didn't know that I could use that ability to lose weight. Delay for a greater purpose. I knew how to do that. A temporary delay for a future gain. You know how to do it too. You don't lack self-control, you don't lack discipline. You just didn't know that you could accept the feelings you experience instead of fight against them. Wow. In this next exercise, Shelley tells you what weight loss is really all about, and I promise you it's not what you've been told.

~~*~*~*~*~*

Is this path like The Yellow Brick Road? Well, I guess it's very similar! Dorothy had all the power she ever wanted all along and didn't know it. You do too. You have this power to make all of your own decisions that will take you to the destination you desire. The Yellow Brick Road took Dorothy to The Emerald City, so she could go home. This path I discovered will take you to a luscious field of green and gold by the riverbank to make it your home. You have the power right now to get there.

Step 2 – TRUTH

Shh... The Truth to Weight Loss is Simple Math

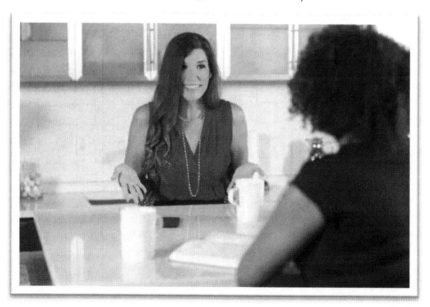

Shelley: I like to draw three rectangles, so you can see we are talking about three separate and independent categories. And those are important words—*separate* and *independent*.

The first category is **Nutrition**. The second category is **Fitness**, and the third category is **Weight**. These three categories can help each other, but they are separate and independent, and I'm going to show you how and why.

Nutrition has to do with the science of how the components of food affect the health of your body. Health is the key word here. Ask yourself why do you or why do you not go to the doctor? Do you have high blood pressure, high cholesterol, high blood sugar? This has to do with the vitamins, minerals, proteins, fats, carbohydrates, etc. and how the science of food affects the health of your body.

Fitness is your exercise. I want you to think of fitness as the performance of your body. *Performance.* How can you make your body perform? How high can you jump? How far can you run? How long can you dance? How much weight can you lift? Fitness is about the strength, flexibility and endurance of your body. This is separate from the other categories.

Weight. When you look at the scale, what do you see?

Participant: Something I don't like.

Shelley: But literally, what do you see?

Participant: A number.

Shelley: Correct. A number. Guess what? The symbol for number is also the symbol for pound, because a pound is a number! **(#)**

By definition, the fact that it's a number means it can be mathematically manipulated. Whether your weight goes up or whether your weight goes down, it's math. That means you can add to it or subtract from it using math.

Controlling your weight is 100% math. That's right. It's pure math. It is <u>100% math</u>.

I want to give you some examples of how these three categories are so different because we have believed that if we want to lose weight, we must focus on our fitness and nutrition.

Has anyone here ever focused on their fitness to lose weight?

(Participants raise hands)

Shelley: Then why are you here?

Participant: It didn't work.

Shelley: What about your nutrition? Who has focused on their nutrition to lose weight?

(Participants raise hands)

Shelley: Then why are you here?

Participant: I'm trying to lose weight, of course.

Shelley: This is what the diet industry tells us, to focus on our fitness and nutrition and we'll lose weight. Here are my examples to help you understand how separate and independent these three categories are.

I happen to know people with very *poor* nutrition, losing weight in hospital beds right now. They're sick, with poor nutrition, losing weight because of math!

When I was 220 pounds and playing tennis, my body could perform, but I couldn't lose weight. Fitness didn't equal weight loss because I was not manipulating the math.

I like to do Zumba for my fitness, and I stand next to a woman who is 40 pounds overweight. She's been 40 pounds overweight for the last seven years that I've known her. She does Zumba, CrossFit, Krav Maga, all sorts of stuff. She is more fit than I, she works her body *more* than me, but she's overweight and I'm not.

Let's talk about your weight now. It is 100% math. Again, I want you to remember that you look down at the scale and you see a number. If you saw a color, you could create art. If you saw a letter, you could write a word. But you don't, you see a number.

Every time you look at that number, I want you to remember that means you can mathematically manipulate it! That's exciting! It is 100% math. Only math. But then again, I like to hold this up (Shelley's before & after 90 lb. weight loss photos) and say, "But don't listen to me."

So *why,* if this is true, *why* have you been deceived for years by the diet industry into believing it's all about your nutrition and fitness?

Shelley (pointing to Nutrition category): *I'll tell you why*! I've got some protein bars to sell you! And shakes! Special meal plans and supplements!

(Pointing to Fitness category): And gym memberships! Fitness routines! Exercise equipment!

(Pointing to Weight category): And… um… um…nothin', I got nothin'… I don't own math. *Nobody* owns math. Anyone can do math.

Now pay no attention to that man behind the curtain.
(Pointing to Nutrition category): "Back to supplements! Cha-ching!! YES! Supplements!!"

This is why, ladies. It's the almighty dollar. This is a multi-*billion-dollar* industry. If they told you the truth, that you could do this all by yourself, that you don't need their product, you wouldn't buy it.

They don't want you to know the truth. Although you're all very smart and educated, so I think you all do know this.

NUTRITION	FITNESS	WEIGHT
The Science of Food	Exercise	# lb.
Vitamins + Minerals = HEALTH	PERFORMANCE Strength Flexibility Endurance	100% MATH 3500 calories = 1 pound

I'm going to tell you another little weight loss secret here, that you'll probably only hear at Losing Coach®.

Many years ago, there was a brilliant scientist. He discovered this thing. And I usually whisper this because it's a bit politically incorrect. He discovered a unit of energy found in food. Do you know what that unit is called?

Participant: Calorie.

Shelley: Yes! Shh… Yes! He discovered a unit of energy called a calorie. And what he discovered is 3500 calories equal one pound. Whether your weight goes up or whether your weight goes down, 3500 calories = one pound. If you have a surplus of 3500 calories, you gain 1 pound. If you have a deficit of 3500 calories, you lose a pound. No matter where those calories come from, regardless of the nutrition, regardless if those calories are salads or Twinkies, if you create a deficit of 3500 calories, you lose a pound. If you have a surplus of 3500 calories, you gain a pound.

Do you know what that means?

That means the only reason you are overweight at all is because you have accumulated a surplus of calories over time.

That's it.

It's that simple. There is no other reason you are overweight.

You didn't make bad choices, you're not stupid, you're not lazy, you're not undisciplined, you do not lack self-control. Nobody here lacks self-control. The only reason you are overweight at all is from the accumulation of the surplus of calories over time.

You were simply unaware of this.

I was playing tennis and trying to eat healthy and I had no awareness of this. And so, I accumulated a surplus of calories over time.

No one here gained all their weight in one day, right? It was accumulated over time and it was simple, simple math.

Listen to me, you haven't done anything wrong! Again, you are not lazy, you are not undisciplined, you do not lack self-control. Math is the only reason. The *only* reason. So, all you have to do is manipulate the math.

~~*~*~*~*

This is solid. Solid truth. I walked on this solid ground. I could see the clearing, I could see this luscious field of green and gold.

Truth is solid. It always is. Always will be. It's not going to change. Solid ground. *This* was the path out.

I stepped onto it. It led me to the field of green and gold by the riverbank.

Solid. Simple. Truth. Math.

~~*~*~*~*~*

Erin: Wow. Math? I can do math. Simple kindergarten math. Everything you ever needed to know about weight loss you learned in kindergarten! I spent years focusing on my fitness. What about you? I spent years improving my nutrition. Can you relate? No wonder I couldn't easily lose weight. I was putting all of my energy into everything but the math.

Understand that weight loss is only about math and you remove the confusion and relieve yourself of feeling overwhelmed. Because you can do simple math. Weight loss is only controlled by math. Believe this truth and you can lose as much weight as you want, whenever you want. Shelley's weight loss is so inspiring because of how big the odds were against her. Do you feel the odds are against you and that they're too great to lose weight? Maybe some inspiration would help you.

Step 3 – LOVE

Remove the Judgement, Restore the Love

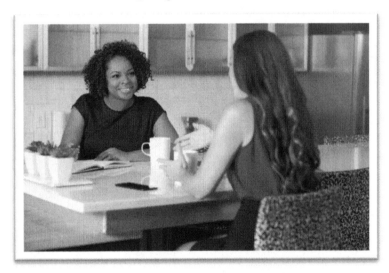

What you'll read next is a bit more of my story, as well as some testimonials from other women who have learned how to lose weight with the Losing Coach process.

~~*~*~*~*~*

Participant A: I thought that I couldn't lose the weight either. But after working with Shelley, I have been able to lose the weight and keep the weight off. I also have gained confidence and I was surprised at how easily the program worked for me.

Part of the main reason that I have the hope that I do, is Shelley has lived this for many years and kept the weight off. That's a true inspiration. Shelley has an insatiable motivational personality that you can just grab onto and you can hold onto it until you can feel it yourself. And by having that available to you, it really does help you to get past any plateaus or walls you're hitting.

Participant B: When Shelley asked me: "Do you want me to help you lose weight?" I said no, I'm really tired of failing. I'm really tired of feeling like a failure. I've wanted to be this person all my life and Shelley was the one person who said you can be. And if you'll take my hand, I'll show you how to do it.

~~*~*~*~*~*

It's just math. That's the truth. And you're probably saying well duh, common-sense, right? But you're wondering why you haven't been able to put this into practice for yourself. What's the secret that all Losing Coach clients know, and what's the magic to the Losing Coach process that gives women this powerful and permanent ability to lose weight for themselves?

Here it is.

First, I want you to find a memory. Excluding all romantic relationships, I want you to think of someone you have done something life-giving, life-changing or life-sustaining for. A child, a pet, a parent. Who have you given birth to, rescued, or sacrificed for?

I want you to go back in time. Whether back in time is forty days, forty weeks, or forty years ago. Go back in time and identify one person who have you given care, comfort, provision and protection to? Who have you given birth to, rescued or sacrificed for?

Did you give birth to your baby? Remember the labor, holding them in your arms, feeding them for the first time? Or did you rescue an animal? Remember taking them into your home, focusing on their needs, gathering everything they needed?

Or did you care for an ill parent? Remember dropping everything? Sitting long hours by their side and feeling the experience of their pain?

Think of how you sacrificially gave care, comfort, provision and protection to them. Think of the very first thing you did for them. What did you do for them? And *why* did you do it?

Why did you feed your baby?

Why did you take them into your home?

Why did you sacrifice your life for theirs?

It wasn't because it's what you were supposed to do. It wasn't because you had to. It was because of LOVE.

LOVE. LOVE is what gave you the power to do everything. LOVE is what gave you the energy to stay up sleepless nights, create a home of warmth and comfort, and sacrifice your life for theirs. LOVE always cares, comforts, provides, and protects.

I'm talking about that real raw emotion of LOVE. Not love as a decision, because if love was a decision, you'd be using your brain and your logic, and we previously talked about using your brain to make decisions.

No, I'm talking about the real raw emotion of LOVE that uses no logic and makes absolutely no sense at all! It doesn't make any sense why you would sacrifice your time, your body, maybe even your life, for someone at the time that could do absolutely nothing for you! Because you see, at the moments that you created life, rescued life, or sustained life, you manifested the LOVE of God.

LOVE is the only thing capable of giving you the power to do what you did.

LOVE is the most powerful energy source of the entire universe!

It is an energy source, just like electricity is an energy source. We plug in this lamp over here into the outlet to access the energy of electricity to give it power to light up.

We are going to plug into the most powerful energy source of the entire universe, this LOVE that can care, comfort, provide and protect *you*! Let's talk about this LOVE and how you can access it for yourself.

What has happened to this LOVE that would have protected you?

Because even though you may not have been aware of the surplus of calories accumulated over time, you knew you were gaining weight. You could see it in the mirror, you could feel it in your clothing. So, what happened to the LOVE that would protect you from that? That wouldn't let this happen to you? Well, here's what happened.

Someone once said to me, "Shelley, you have a very white heart." I asked him, "What does that mean?" He said, "It means you're good, you're honest, you're pure. Your heart is full of LOVE."

I believe we are all born with a white heart. We are all born with a heart full of LOVE. You are good, you are honest and pure. But what has happened over time in our lives are these arrows that have hit your white heart. These arrows are the insults and the injuries of life. They are abuse, mistreatment, abandonment, neglect, and sometimes tragic and unfortunate events that are nobody's fault. They come from our friends, our family, and those who love us very much!

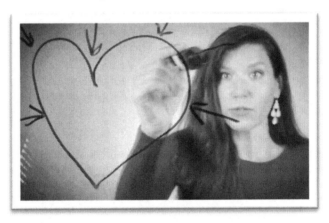

I'm going to sum up twenty, thirty, maybe forty years of your life.

And as these arrows hit your heart, it starts to look like this. (Shelley starts to color in the heart with a black marker.)

"He's so mad at me, I must've done something wrong!"

"She criticizes everything that I do!"

"I'm not as pretty as her so she must be better than me!"

"If I'd only worked harder, I'd be farther along by now!"

"I'm not sure he even loves me!"

"Oh, I failed there!"

"Now I think she hates me!!"

"This is all my fault!"

"You know I don't know if he ever loved me and really what's there to love anymore?!"

"If I hadn't done that, we wouldn't be having all these problems!"

"They wouldn't be suffering right now if I hadn't done that!"

"I don't know how I ended up here!"

"I'm so fat and pathetic!"

"Life wasn't supposed to turn out like this!"

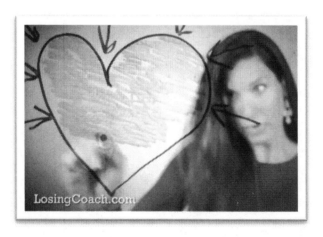

And life wasn't supposed to turn out like this...

That's all that's happened. These arrows have hit, and you've absorbed everything as your fault.

But see, the LOVE is still there. (Pointing to white area in the heart) It's just been crowded out by the absorption of judgement.

And so, to restore the LOVE…

We need to erase the judgement. And it starts to look like this…

"Actually, he loves you very much."

"She never meant to hurt you."

"You are very beautiful."

"You are good enough."

"You worked really hard and you did the best you knew how to do at the time."

"Actually, he still loves you, he's always loved you and he didn't mean to hurt you."

"That was not your fault."

"You didn't cause anyone's suffering."

"You didn't do anything wrong."

"You haven't done anything wrong."

It's that simple. Erase the judgement and you restore the LOVE.

You haven't done anything wrong.

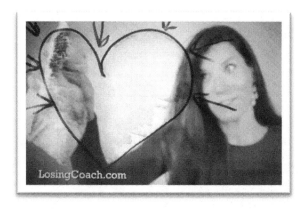

Listen to me. I'll say it again, you haven't done anything wrong! Remove the judgement and you restore the LOVE. This is the LOVE that will protect you, the LOVE that will empower you to do this for yourself. You've already done it for others. Now is the time for you to do it for yourself!

You are good, and pure, and this is my message to help every woman lose weight. I am bringing you the message of salvation to weight loss. Remove the judgement and restore the LOVE. You haven't done anything wrong.

LOVE.

What I learned and what changed me forever was this LOVE.

~~*~*~*~*~*

The seed of LOVE. I removed the judgement, and the seed of LOVE implanted itself in me right there by the riverbank in the luscious field of green and gold.

And so there I was, now fertilized with this seed, implanted in me to restore all the LOVE I needed.

What was the seed of LOVE? The voice that spoke quietly and gently, not with logic, but with *feeling,* real, raw, emotional *feeling* that I was LOVED. I was cared for, and comforted. I was provided for. I was protected.

Now I was safe; now I was home.

On solid ground, fertilized with LOVE, a new life emerged. I could now plant my roots. I could grow. I could flourish. All from one seed of LOVE. And from one seed came forth a tree.

A very strong tree, like a giant oak. Not a tree that would wither, not a tree that would fall down in the storms, a tree that would last forever, a tree of life. And only the seed of LOVE can create a tree of life.

And there I was! With Power, Truth & LOVE. A tree of life! Not only that, but a svelte, healthy, 130 lb. tree, just like I wanted to be.

You've just experienced it. Steps 1, 2, & 3—Power, Truth & LOVE.

The Truth About Weight Loss
Power, Truth and LOVE! Worksheet

1. A word or two that describes how I feel right now:

2. My weight today:

3. Power—The infinite power of God inside of you to bring about the desires of your heart. Describe how you have the ability to make your own decisions.

4. Do you understand that you can make decisions to bring about your desires based on what you believe, what you know, and how you react?

5. Can you embrace your belief that there is a greater purpose to your decisions and accept that your feelings are involuntary reactions to your experiences, while telling yourself what you know to be true? (Delay, Never Deprivation)

6. Truth—What did you learn about the difference between Nutrition, Fitness and Weight Loss? (Weight Loss is ONLY MATH)

7. LOVE—LOVE cares, comforts, provides, and protects. Did you go back in time and identify someone you have already given this to? WHY you gave them everything is because of LOVE. How much do you LOVE them? (The most powerful energy source of the entire universe is LOVE)

8. What kinds of thoughts and feelings did you experience as you read through Steps 1 through 3, The Truth About Weight Loss? Please elaborate on all you are feeling right now.

www.losingcoach.com

Step 4 – FAITH

Giving Voice to Your Higher Purpose

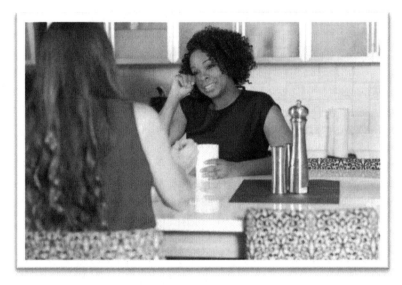

I f you have not completed writing your Letter to God, please do so before you read this chapter.

Instructions for writing your Letter to God are in the "Get Set" chapter called Articulate Your Higher Purpose.

Today you get a chance to express your personal FAITH by

reading your Letter to God. Whoever you have written this letter to, you need to express it out loud.

Be in a private, quiet place right now.

Stop and read your Letter to God out loud. Literally read it out loud.

This is one of the most powerful moments in our process, so be sure to pause reading this book and read your letter out loud.

Now pause. Read your letter to God out loud right now.

Then, come back.

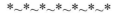

Reading Your Letter to God

Now take a look at your reflection in the mirror.

That woman you see...she's asking to be heard.

In a gentle, kind, quiet voice, she's simply asking for you to listen to her.

How did that feel to read your letter out loud? Was it emotional for you?

Now I want you to total up all the years you've been trapped by your weight. How many years all together have you struggled with your weight?

Now I want you to imagine you've literally been in a prison for all those years, and all those years, your voice was silenced. Nobody cared what you wanted, how you felt, or what you wanted to do. You were confined by the prison rules and the prison walls. You couldn't even see the outside world. You were confined to a cell all alone and were never free to come and go as you please.

Now imagine, after all those years, you are finally released!

On your release day, you are finally free to go *wherever* and *whenever* you please. You are no longer confined by rules, or walls, and you are *free*! Free to express what *you* really want, and how *you* really feel, and what *you* want to do.

And you've written it all down in a letter to God, and you've traveled through the open wilderness, to the top of a mountain, and standing on top of this mountain, you read this letter to God out loud.

You're hearing your voice, for the *first time*, express what *you* want, how *you* feel, and what *you* want to do.

You're also remembering what it felt like to not have a voice, to not be heard, to not have hope, and to not have a future.

You realize you almost gave up a number of times, while imprisoned, but you didn't! Your tears indicate you realize you were that despondent, you were that hopeless.

And now you're free and have faith in a future that can come true, and a dream that can really come true.

YOU ARE FREE!

Next, I talk with a client after she read her letter to God out loud to me.

~~*~*~*~*~*

Shelley: Now let me ask you, how much weight have you lost this first week?

Client: 7 pounds.

Shelley: Okay. Now let's pretend, God forbid, you leave my office here today, and as you're driving home, you get killed in a car accident. What would this 7 pounds mean?

Client: (hesitating)...Nothing?

Shelley: That's right, if you died today, this 7 pounds that you just lost would mean absolutely NOTHING. Nothing...

Client: Right.

Shelley: I know what you're thinking, but you don't want to say it. You're like, "Why is my weight loss coach telling me my weight loss means nothing?"

Client: Right.

Shelley: Again, listen, if you died in a car accident today, these seven pounds would mean absolutely nothing.

What you just articulated in that letter to God, this is your **faith**.

This is your faith that your life will *continue*, and that this weight loss will mean something!

Now, I know that song, "Live Like You're Dying", it's a very romantic song. But we don't actually live that way. Because if you die today, it means nothing.

We tend to talk about faith as it applies to religion, or the afterlife. What I'm speaking of is your very *practical faith*, faith that your life will continue, and your weight loss will mean something.

Because seriously, if you're going to die today, it really does mean nothing. And if you're going to die tomorrow... Let me tell you something, even if you don't die today and you die tomorrow, please don't do this! Please, let it go and forget about it.

If someone had a crystal ball and told me that tomorrow is my time, it's simply my time to go, already written in the book of life and death, and there's nothing I can do about it, and I die tomorrow, listen, I'm not going to concern myself with another calorie whatsoever!

If I'm going to die tomorrow, guess what I'm going to do? I'm going to eat it up, drink it up, and sex it up all I can tonight! (laughter)

But see, we actually don't live like that. We live by *faith* that our actions today actually have consequences for tomorrow. Be it for good or for bad. That's why we don't live like we're dying.

Let me say it again, "And now you're free, and have *faith* in a future that can come true!" So now you are free, and you have expressed your faith to God.

This means something.

Last week, we talked about your greater purpose in step one, Power, in the decision-making analysis, and we were implying it was your weight loss, and indeed, your greater purpose is your weight loss!

Your faith in the *meaning* of your weight loss is now your greater purpose to your greater purpose!

Understand how meaningful this is for you! This is your faith. You've just articulated it.

This is for your son. This is so you can enjoy a healthy relationship with your partner. This is so you can have a *life*!

There is nothing shallow about what you're doing here. This is very meaningful for you.

This is your purpose. Read it again whenever you must be reminded of it.

Client: Okay.

Shelley: Okay? Begin to have this nice, honest, expressive relationship with yourself.

Client: Right.

Shelley: Honestly, because this is *you* helping *you*. You are helping yourself now, so have an honest, expressive relationship with yourself. That's what you did!

You got to hear it for the first time, and it was honest, real, and it was meaningful. This is pivotal in the process.

Again, you don't have to ruminate in the past, but look at what you just expressed. This is *your* expression. Your true, honest, real, raw expression to the divine of what you want. You believe in God, or a higher power, correct?

Client: Mm-hmm (affirmative).

Shelley: The divine heard you. He heard you and He's going to give you all the desires of your heart, because you deserve it. You deserve it! You haven't done anything wrong. You've been pure. You've been good. You've been LOVE. You deserve to be blessed now. The divine heard you, and the divine will answer you.

~~*~*~*~*~*

Imagine praying for rain during a drought. You look up a lot.

You look up until it comes.

Hearing my voice and expressing my faith in this letter to God, in the open wilderness on top of a mountain, was me looking up. Looking up with certainty in my greater purpose, until the skies opened up and poured down on my tree with water that would fill up the river it was planted next to, to give me all the nourishment I needed.

Step 5 – HOPE

Setting Short Term Goals - The Hope Chart

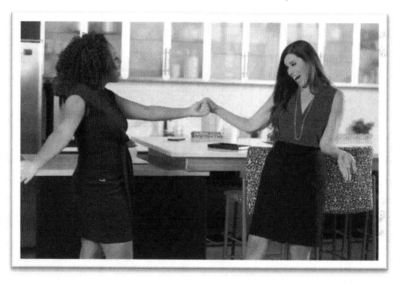

Here is the next step after FAITH. This is HOPE.
As you have experienced, POWER, TRUTH, and LOVE will give you immediate weight loss.

FAITH is understanding the meaning and greater purpose to it.

Now you will learn that HOPE does not disappoint, and it will carry you forward to reach your goals.

This Hope Chart is looking at your immediate future, looking at some short-term goals for the next 8-12 weeks ahead of you.

Understand when I began at 220 lbs., never in a million years did I ever dream about being close to 130 lbs. or competing in the Mrs. Ohio pageant, or being who I am today.

I started dreaming and hoping about losing a few pounds. I looked at my immediate future and began with short-term goals.

After you read about The Hope Chart, make extra copies for yourself, then complete your chart.

The Hope Chart

Next is a conversation between me and a client as we plan the client's short-term weight loss goals. This is included to give you a sense of the thought process behind The Hope Chart. You don't need to worry about the details of this particular client's goals, it's just to give an example of how you'll want to think through your own chart.

~~*~*~*~*~*

Shelley: We're going to map out some of your future short-term goals.

These are always short-term goals.

The date today is May 18th, and today you're 158.8. Now, what we want to do on this chart is we can work forward, or we can work backwards. Each line represents one week.

I want you to think of an upcoming *thing* for yourself, some special event, a birthday, anniversary, a celebration, something important to you within the next 10 weeks. It doesn't have to be in 10 weeks. It can be in six weeks, seven weeks. Is there anything coming up for you?

Client: My anniversary is September 27th.

Shelley: And what would you like to weigh on your anniversary?

Client: I'd like to be at my goal weight, but I don't know if that's doable.

Shelley: Well, it's in four months.

Client: Okay. So, 135?

Shelley: Great! 135. We're going to work backwards from that. Write 135 on the bottom line.

Client: I can count the weeks if you want me to.

Shelley: Yeah. June, July, August, September. It's four months. That would be 16 weeks?

Client: It's going to be more than that. September 27th is a Sunday.

Shelley: Okay. Then we'll map this out every two weeks. We're going to make every line here, two weeks.

Client: Okay.

Shelley: We'll work backwards, so we'll do September 13th on that line above the bottom.

Client: It's 18 weeks.

Shelley: Great. Then we'll start with two weeks before your anniversary. So, if you want to be 135 on your anniversary, let's say two weeks before, you are 138? We're working backwards.

Let's fill in all of the dates first.

Client: Okay (writes down the dates in 2-week increments)

Shelley: Great! See how we're putting the dates like that! We go from May 25th... to September 20th! So now again, we can work forwards and backwards. Let's now go to the top.

What do you want to be in seven days, on May 25th? You're 158.8 today.

Client: I'd like to shoot for 156.

Shelley: Yeah, 156. Great. Then June 8th, would then be two weeks after 156. In two weeks, you could be 153?

Client: Yeah.

Shelley: Two weeks after that? Could maybe be 150? That would be three pounds over two weeks.

July 6th, two weeks after that? You got plenty of time here. So, you can start slowing down. Let's say two pounds over that two weeks?

Client: Okay, 148.

Shelley: Uh-huh. Then July 20th, July 6th through July 20th...

As you create this hope chart, what do you need to be aware of over this week or this time period? What do you have planned? What's going on?

Is that going to be a slow time for you? Are you vacationing? Anything like that?

Client: Not that I know of.

Shelley: Okay. From July 6th to July 20th, we can go forward again, and keep filling this in, 146, 144, 142, 140...

So, we got May 25th, 156. You can do that in this next coming week. That's 2.8 pounds. You're on a roll, you're riding the momentum of the very quick weight loss in the beginning. We're aware that it's probably going to slow down, so we're going to respect that as well.

Then June 8th, we've got 153. Again, these are two-week increments, so we're going down three pounds every two weeks. June 22nd is 150. July 6th is 148. July 20th is 146. August 3rd, 144. August 17th, 142. August 31st, 140. September 13th, 138. September 27th, 135.

Now do you see it?

Client: Yeah.

Shelley: You see what you can accomplish?

Client: Doable.

Shelley: Yep! How's that make you feel?

Client: Good.

Shelley: Now, this is what I want you to do. I want you to see it. See how possible it is for you to be 135 by your anniversary. We've got your weight loss even slowing down. We've got you taking your time. You may surpass these goals. You may reach half of them. If you are not 135, but say, 141.6 on your anniversary, are you going to be upset?

Client: No.

Shelley: Okay. I want you to take this other blank copy of the chart home and I want you to make copies of this. Because at any point, if next week you come back here, on May 25th and you are not 156, if you are 157, if you are 155.8, we're going to take this hope chart and we're going to throw it away!
(Shelley rips up the hope chart just created and throws it in the trash.)

It's just a piece of paper.

So, I want you to throw that away at any point! Start over! If you reach half your goals, if you surpass your goals, I want you to throw that away, it's just a piece of paper! And I want you to start over.

Client: Okay.

Shelley: Okay? Because it's going to change. You're not going to hit those numbers on those dates. You're going to hit them sooner or later. It's not a matter of if, it's a matter of when.

This is for your vision! This is for you to see it's possible. If you do not reach them at the specific date that you specified, throw that paper away! If you're short on paper, I'll give you more paper. (laughing) Make copies of that... (blank hope chart)

This is not to hold you to it. Throw this away at any point in time. I did this all the time. All. the. time. (create hope charts, throw away, start over and create another one!)

You know why I did it all the time?

Because I *never reached my goals*!

Listen to me. (Holding up her Before & After photos): I. Never. Reached. My. Goals.

Look at my photos. *I never reached my goals!*

I'd reach half. I would reach half of my goal, and then I'd start over! And I'd reach half again and then I'd start over again. Do you know what happens when you reach half and start over? And reach half and start over? You get there!

It's like I'm trying to drive from here to California at 100 miles per hour, but I'm only driving 50 miles per hour. I still get there. I *still* get there!

This is for you to see you can be 135 by your anniversary. But if you're 140, you'll take it!

Client: I won't be mad. (smiling)

Shelley: You won't be mad!

So, this is our hope chart. This is step five, hope. These are our short-term goals that we do every week actually.

Always have short term goals! Even in my maintenance, I have short term goals. Because if I'm not always trying, always reaching for something, guess what happens to my weight? It slowly creeps back up.

So, I constantly always have a number in my mind. Always!

Even if I'm at my goal, I have it in my mind. It's something I want to continue to see.

It's kind of like your business. Everything that you do, if you want to achieve financial success and you achieve it, then what do you want to do with the wealth you've earned? You want to keep it, you don't want to lose it! You've worked hard for it. So, it's there in your mind. You're aware of it. You're not obsessed with it. You're aware of it.

You always have a vision for the future of what you want to accomplish next. That's what this is. It's not often like this [gestures smooth descent]. It looks like this. Always up and down. That's what you're going to see with your weight, but you're going to keep on keeping on and you're going to accumulate the success that you desire.

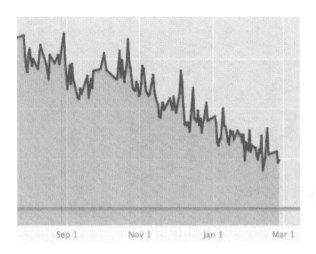

Sep 1   Nov 1   Jan 1   Mar 1

So great. We've got the hope chart.

(Next Shelley talks with another client about her four-page Hope Chart that she completed at home and brought back with her to her next session with Shelley.)

Shelley: Great, now let's just say, you come back here on May 15th, and you have your goal as 211.6, but you don't reach that goal.

Client: So low. I haven't seen that number for a very, very long time.

Shelley: Here's what I want you to do. Did you make copies?

Client: Oh, you mean extra blank copies? Yes.

Shelley: Good, Good, Good. Basically, what I'm going to do (Crumples page 1), what I want you to do (crumples page 2), is

I want you to start over! (crumples page 3) This is what I want you to do at any point along the way. (crumples page 4)

Client: (Gasps) (Laughs) Okay.

Shelley: All right. I didn't get a chance to do that with you last week. Because I gave it to you really quick and said, "Take this home and do it."

Client: It was good homework.

Shelley: Did that shock you? (referring to crumpling up the chart) That's a shock factor there.

Client: A little bit!

Shelley: Yes. It's supposed to, because the point is, at any point along the way that you need to do that, you do that. Okay?

Client: Yes.

Shelley: All right. Start over. Actually, if you want, use this (uncrumples chart) because I know you did some serious calculations with this…. (hands back chart)

Do you know how many times I created charts for myself? About every other day. Okay? I would do this, keep doing it. I didn't rip that up to say don't do that. I ripped it up to say do it *again*! Start over as many times as you need to, because what if Mother's Day comes and you're not down to 211.5? You're going to look at your chart and go, "Oh. I screwed up."

Nope. No, you didn't. It's just paper. Really, it's just paper. We have trash cans. You have trash cans, right?

Client: Yes.

Shelley: You have plenty of paper at home?

Client: Yep.

Shelley: Okay! I want you to rip that up! And I didn't expect you to come back with four pieces of paper! (laughter)

Client: I was the kid that sat in the front of the classroom, right?

Shelley: And that's the point ... I want you to stay front and center and *do this*! Do your hope chart. The point is start over whenever. Rip it up. Throw it away. That's why I said make copies, whenever you need to.

You know why you might rip it up? Because you surpassed your goal. Okay? You may rip it up because you *surpass* your goal! You may rip it up because you missed half your goal; you got halfway there. Rip it up and start over. It's a very powerful thing to do.

We get so *attached* to "I've got to do this, and I've got to do it now." Listen, I'm a big believer in goals! That's why we set them each week. But you better let them go as quickly as they come. If you want to reach your final destination, then let it go! Because if you hold onto one specific goal, and you don't get there, you don't reach it, you say, "I've screwed up!" and in floods the judgement again. It's *just* paper!

So, if you don't reach your goals, there's nothing wrong with you. I know, because I did this. You don't have to listen to me, but I'm telling you what I did.

I used my journal to create my hope charts. I actually didn't use a separate piece of paper. I simply used my journal.

And I would usually go out four to six weeks. In four to six weeks, what do I want to see?

This is what I want to see... but then... I wouldn't get there.
And then I'd start a new chart, even before that chart was finished.

Start a new chart. What do I want to see? I'm getting my mind wrapped around the next goal and the next part of this journey.

I'm looking at it. I'm embracing it.

Whether I get there in the time that I hoped, is completely irrelevant.

~~*~*~*~*

My hope, my short-term goals, grew a feeling in me that eventually always carried me to my goal.

The branches of my tree were continually reaching, and the more I reached, the longer they grew. Have you ever seen the branches of a giant oak tree? They reach far and wide. Every goal I set grew my branches farther and wider. So, reach! Just reach!

The Hope Chart Worksheet

(Make copies before filling it out!)

Hope for the Near Future!

Today's Date:

Today's Weight:

Date	Goal Weight

Step 6 – SELF CONTROL

Use Journaling to Build Self Control

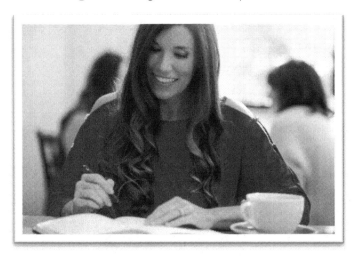

A s you learned, weight loss comes only and always from a caloric deficit.

In an imaginary world, a caloric deficit could easily be created if you were in a cage on a deserted island and the only food you could eat is what was dropped into your cage. In the real world, ensuring you create a caloric deficit is not as automatic.

Journaling is the only way to ensure you create the caloric deficit, otherwise, it's left to chance. Journaling is where you get to CONTROL the number of calories you consume.

Consider yourself the captain, the boss, the supervisor, the director, the project manager, the controller. You're in control. Don't leave it to chance. This is your SELF-CONTROL.

Yes, you can lose weight without journaling. (On that deserted island, no self-control is needed because someone else would be controlling your life. :)) But you're not on that deserted island, so you have to have self-control. And with your JOURNAL—you will!

You are in control now. It doesn't matter what you eat, where you eat, how you eat, when you eat, or with whom you eat.

If you take the time to pay attention, look at a label, look up the calories, measure it, pick up pen and paper and write it down, you are exercising SELF-CONTROL!

Record the number of calories so you can ensure you create the caloric deficit and *you will lose weight*!

This is important. I HIGHLY recommend actual pen and paper for your journaling. Why? Because I've coached a few women who were trying to do everything right with counting and measuring and having no success in moving the number on the scale. Each and every time, it was because they were journaling using an app on their phone. As soon as they switched to paper and pen, they saw the weight loss they desired.

Not only do apps for journaling seem to be a roadblock (although you can use the app for looking up calories, that's fine, but not for your actual recording and keeping track of your calories), but they also try to "grade" you and we don't need that judgement!

They can also complicate the formula by calculating calories burned in exercise. Do NOT do this.

Why? Because we are keeping it simple by only tracking your intake in calories. It's that simple. Sure, if you exercise, are you burning calories? Of course! We will take that as a BONUS to our weight loss! Calculating calories burned in exercise leads to misleading information... really... how do they know you burned 450 calories in an aerobics class? They don't. You don't. Only your body knows, and maybe it actually only burned 398 calories... you really don't know.

Just enjoy eating whatever you want, then JOURNAL it.

Record the number of calories so you can *ensure* you create the caloric deficit and you will lose weight!

Journaling

I was 220 lbs. and decided to count, track, and journal my calories to create a caloric deficit, setting my caloric limit to approximately 1200 calories/day. You can determine your caloric target based on your current weight according to the suggestions offered on the Journaling Worksheet at the end of this chapter.

This is a conversation with a client about how she decided what calorie limit to set for herself and how journaling will help her control how much she eats.

~~*~*~*~*~*

Shelley: It depends how fast you want your weight loss to be.

Client: 1600?

Shelley: Yeah, I'd say 1400 to 1600. You can give yourself a range or you can give yourself a limit, a number limit. It just depends on your current weight.

I was 220, and I did 1200 calories a day. Women that are over 300 pounds may be up into that 1600-1800 range. At 255, I would suggest the 1400 to 1600.

You can, whenever you want to speed up your weight loss and create more of a caloric deficit, go lower, okay?

Client: Okay.

Shelley: Again, it's whatever way you want to do it, it is up to you. I'm just here to help guide and direct and show you what I did, and then you get to decide how you want to put it into practice, okay?

So, what I did was I created in my mind, this image of 1200 calories and I viewed it like, here's the bar [holding her hand up]. Here's the standard, 1200 calories a day. And some days, I went a little bit low, some days I went higher, but basically, I tried to do this.

Client: Right.

Shelley: Okay, because again the math is going to accumulate over time. This is about the accumulation over time. So, when I got up to 1200 calories, I stopped. Again, some days were higher, and that was okay, a lot of grace here, a lot of "perfection-not-required".

Erin gave herself a range of 1200 to 1400 and she went like this [up and down in that range]. Again, maybe some days were high or low, that's okay, whatever works for you. You can give yourself a limit of 1600, 1500, whatever you want, or you can give yourself a range, 1400 to 1600. It doesn't matter. It's going to create the caloric deficit accumulated over time. It's really whatever works best for you, okay?

So, for me, again, I did a 1200 bar that told me, "I'm going to stop at 1200."

I weighed myself every day, and I wrote my weight in the upper-right corner of my journal page. I put the date and my weight.

Now, we want to compare apples to apples every day. This is what I suggest to everyone, "Get up, go pee, get naked, get on the scale," or near naked or whatever. Take your pajamas off.
So, it's: wake up, go pee, get naked, get on the scale, where you're then comparing apples to apples every day. And that pretty much will be your lowest weight of the day.

I don't care how you journal necessarily or what kind of organization you want to put to it, but you want to get the measurement.

You know, was it one cup of mashed potatoes or half a cup of mashed potatoes? And then the calorie count. And just keep track, okay? And then, you can keep a running total. I would get to a stopping point around 1200, and I would just double underline to communicate to my brain, "Stop!"

So now, let me ask you, when you fed your baby formula, or even, say, medicine, the times you had to give your baby medicine, did you measure it or did you half-ass it?

Client: Measure it.

Shelley: Measured it, okay. Take out your measuring spoons and your measuring cups!

Client: Okay.

Shelley: You're going to need to measure, because, again, one cup of mashed potatoes has exactly twice as many calories as half a cup of mashed potatoes, and you're going to serve yourself well to have accuracy. We want accuracy.

We need accuracy. There's no judgement here. I don't care what you eat. There's absolutely no judgement here. I don't care how much you eat.

You are going to be manipulating the math and you're going to need accurate measurements, okay?

Client: Right.

Shelley: So that's it. You can organize it and write it anyway you want. Just on a blank piece of paper in a notebook, we're going to keep track of your calories.

Now, a couple things about that. Again, I told you—measure everything! Accuracy is going to matter.

You're going to have to find a resource for yourself on calorie counts. I checked out a book at the library. That was back in the day. We got the internet, you can use a website, or get an app!

And we'll talk more about the apps, because it's not something that I want you to use for actually journaling in. I want you to do your journal on paper with pen.

Client: Okay.

Shelley: But use the apps to look up calories. That's it. I don't care about sugar, I don't care about fat or carbs, I don't care about any of that. The only thing we're focusing on is calories. Sometimes, when you use the apps, they want to grade you.

Client: Right.

Shelley: Ignore it! I don't care if they grade a food as a D-minus. Ignore it, okay?

And If you record your weight in an app, tomorrow morning, like, if you put your weight in today at 255, and tomorrow morning you're 254, it's going to say, "Whoa, you're losing weight at a dangerously fast pace." Ignore it! Ignore everything that any app, any website, any package has to say, except for calories.

So, when you go shopping, when you see the "light", the "diet", the "low sugar", "low fat", go ahead and turn that package around and see if the calories are lower. The only thing we care about is calories at this point.

Many of those "light" and "non-fat" products *are* lower in calories a lot of the time, so look at them!

I'm not saying, *ignore* low-fat and low-carb items, I'm saying, only be concerned with the calorie count.

I've got suggestions for you if you're a carb person or if you're a bread person. I'm a bread person, I *love* bread! And I almost immediately switched to low-calorie bread, okay?

Client: Okay.

Shelley: My bread is 35 calories a slice.

Client: Mine too.

Shelley: Good. You know, because I'd rather have *two* sandwiches anyways, right? (Laughter) True, true!

I want you to start thinking about satiation for yourself. Satiation, satiating yourself.

You're going to feel hungry because you're going to be decreasing your calorie count, and you'll be able to accept that, but feeling hungry is not the point, that's not what we're trying to do. That's not going to help you, to feel hungry all the time.

We really don't want you to feel hungry. We want you to feel satisfied. We want you to stay satiated. *That* is what's going to help you. So now you have to look at foods that satiate you, okay? Even if the foods that satiate you may not be considered "diet" or "low-calorie". I'm going to give you some examples.

Baked potato. Baked potato gets shamed by the diet world for being this "carb", oh no, it's a "carb", and it's not low calorie, but it's not high calorie, I think it's around 200 calories!

I don't know. It depends on the size of the potato, right? I'm like, "Wait a minute, regardless if it's high or low-calorie, a baked potato fills me up. It satiates my hunger. I'm willing to spend my calories on that!"

Chili. When I go to Wendy's, I always get chili. Chili. Well, their small chili's only 200 calories. I don't care if it has red meat, I don't care if beans are high in calorie. I don't care if it has carbs. I don't care. It's a food that fills me up, so it satiates me. That's a winner!

So, you want to start looking for food that works for you. You're going to discover them. I don't know what they are for you right now. You will discover them for yourself.

Through your journal, you'll learn everything. You're going to look back at your journal, and say, "Hey! When I ate that, I was able to create a nice caloric deficit and not feel hungry. So that's a food that I like! That's a food I want to choose again." Your journal is going to speak so much truth to you. That's where all your learning is going to happen, in that journal.

The other beautiful thing is, the math is the math is the math and it's going to accumulate over time no matter what you do, okay? Here's something very helpful. Your calorie count starts over at zero every day at midnight!

Here's where the delay comes in. It's 10:00 pm at night and you're dying for a snack. Can you delay it for two hours and put it on your next day's journal? Yeah. Your calorie count starts over at zero every day at midnight. So, you can do that!

You may be at 1600 calories for the day and you're done, and your goal is to create a caloric deficit. I would say to you, yes, wait *two* hours and put it on your next day's journal. You can be creative with this!

Remember it's the math accumulated over time? So, we've got Sunday, Monday, Tuesday, Wednesday, etc. If you did this: 1400, 1400, 1400, 1400 every day, that is equal to if you did this: 1200, 1600, 1800, 1000.

It's the same. So, that's where you get permission to have the high and the low variations. Hey, if you go high one day, guess what you can do the next day?

Client: Go low.

Shelley: Yes, you can go *low*! There's never "permanent damage" here. It all can be reversed! That's the beauty of math!

Client: Right.

Shelley: What you add, you can subtract! There's no permanent damage here! So, right, if you go high on one day, go low the next day. You'll be fine!

Client: That's where I usually mess up, because I eat too much and then I...

Shelley: Then you say, "Screw it. I'm done."

Client: Yeah, exactly.

Shelley: I know.

Client: Might as well keep going!

Shelley: Right? That's why the whole idea of, "Well, guess I'll keep eating and just start my diet Monday."

No... even if it's Saturday night, the math will still be accumulating, because this math always accumulates.

I mean, it's like saying, "I'm cleaning my house on Monday, so I'll go ahead and throw things all around and purposely make it more messy right now." You're just giving yourself more work to do in the future. That's *crazy*! I don't purposely mess up my house more because I don't want to clean it right now. I'm aware that the mess will accumulate.

Understand you can manipulate the math however you want, but it's all going to be accumulative.

You've got the power to delay.

It's simply saying, "I know I will eat later. So, I don't have to eat right now. I'm going to accept feeling hungry."

And I told you, if you're going to lose weight, you're going to feel hungry at times. It's a big secret in real weight loss. But nobody wants you to know that! I'm telling you now... be prepared... you *will* feel hungry at times and you'll be okay!

Nobody wants you to know that... because, again, if you knew that, you wouldn't buy their product that's advertising you can lose weight and not feel hungry. It's a lie. Nobody wants you to know if you're going to lose weight, you're going to feel hungry! And I'm here to tell you if you're going to lose weight, there's going to be times you're going to feel hungry! But you're going to be able to accept it!

Because again, it's going to be about delay, and you will say to yourself, "It's 3:00. I'm hungry, but I can accept that

because I'm eating dinner at 5:00. I'm okay, I'm okay. I'm not dying. I'm totally okay!"

Let me give you an example now of how making these low-calorie substitutes can help you.

Again, when you go to the grocery store, I want you to turn everything around and look at the label now. I want you to look at the packages, look at the cans, look at everything that you're buying.

I had a client. She was very young. She's 19 years old, and her mother asked if she could come to her sessions with her because she was so young, and I said, "Sure, I don't mind. Your mom can come." She was very supportive.

My young client *loved* the program! I mean, she lost 25 pounds.

She's actually now a professional cheerleader. She loved the program! She was so happy! She kept saying, "This is a happy program. I love it!"

So, her mom used to make her grilled cheese sandwiches for lunch. Did your mom ever make grilled cheese sandwiches? Yeah, me too. And it was never just *one* grilled cheese sandwich; it was always two, right? Same thing for this girl. Her mom would make her two grilled cheese sandwiches for lunch.

So, before she did this process, we're looking at her lunch. Okay. An average slice of white bread is 80 calories. That is, when you buy regular bread, you're looking at 80 calories a slice. So, it's 160 calories for each sandwich. A slice of American cheese is 100 calories. And of course, they're just slapping on the butter, and who knows how much, because they're not measuring it, but that was maybe 100 calories, could be more.

Each sandwich is 360 calories. So, her lunch is 720 calories in two sandwiches, and that's even before the tomato soup!

After beginning this process, she said, "I still want two grilled cheese sandwiches for lunch." That's what she liked, that's what she wanted. So here's what she did.

She switched to a low-calorie bread. Okay, 35 calories a slice, so that's 70 calories for each sandwich.

She found this cheese that Kraft makes, a low-calorie cheese, it's 25 calories a slice. I didn't even know about it. I bought it. I tried it. It's maybe not considered "nutritious" and it's maybe not that tasty by itself, but melted on the sandwich, it actually was just fine. She just wanted melted cheese on her grilled cheese sandwich, right? So, it's 25 calories a slice.

And she used zero-calorie spray butter. Again, is it nutritious? Not for me to say, but maybe neither is butter, so zero calories for this zero-calorie spray butter.

Now each sandwich is 95 calories! She turned a 720-calorie lunch into 190 calories by finding low-calorie substitutes for the foods that she like to eat!

She didn't feel deprived and she was happy! This 720 calories was probably no more nutritious than this 190 calories. She was happy. She liked it. She lost weight. That's what that looks like. It's very simple. So we want to look for low-calorie substitutes.

And we want to exercise *delay*.

We want to measure, because maybe we only want half a serving, because we want to save some calories. So, measuring, counting the calories and limiting what you take in is what we're doing.

But again, there's no judgement. Your journal's going to speak to you, and you'll be able to decide for yourself what you want to eat and how much you want to eat.

Paper-pen journaling is required, even if you use an app to look up calories. There's a connection with the brain with writing it out; it's going to decrease your appetite. It will be a slow process of your appetite decreasing that you won't see right away but trust me. You write in your journal every day. You journal your calories every day, no judgement. You just keep doing that.

You're decreasing your appetite by the mere act of doing that, and that's what you want!

Weight loss is very difficult with an increased appetite. Weight loss is very easy with a decreased appetite! So, do the process, write in the journal. It will decrease your appetite, and that's what you want!

It will also help you ensure you are creating the caloric deficit and achieving the weight loss you desire right now.

Here is a quick glance at two different versions of journaling, one reflecting truth and accuracy, and one not. See the difference between what someone might journal "loosely", forgetting things, assuming some things have no calories, and not measuring, versus what the body actually consumes and processes.

Journaling TRUTH

Loose	Estimated Calories
Lite English Muffin	100
Egg	70
Nature Valley bar	130
Grapes	0
Carrots	0
Ham sandwich (70+60)	130
Potato Chips	160
Banana	105
Southwest Chicken Strips	140
Medium Baked Potato	160
1 Tbsp Sour Cream	30
Green Salad	0
Salad dressing	80
Dinner Roll	110
Total	1215

True & Concise	Accurate Calories
Lite English Muffin	100
Egg	70
8 oz. Orange Juice	110
Fish oil supplement	15
Sweet & Salty almond bar	160
Grapes, 1 cup	62
3 medium carrots	75
Bread	70
6 slices of ham	80
1 Tbsp Mayonnaise	90
1.5 Oz Potato chips	240
Large banana	125
5 oz. Southwest Chicken Strips	183
Large Baked Potato	280
1.5 Tbsp Sour Cream	45
I ½ cup Green Salad	33
Salad dressing	92
Dinner Roll	110
Wine, 1 glass	165
5 Crackers	77
Total	2182

See the difference in the total calorie count? Accuracy matters.

If you think you have consumed 1200 calories in a day because you have journaled "loosely", yet your body knows it actually consumed closer to 2200 calories, you will not lose weight, you won't believe in the math, and you will be left feeling very frustrated and wanting to throw in the towel.

Here are a REAL CLIENT's numbers her first week of journaling with truth and accuracy:

Date	Weight	Calories
9/20	216.5	1352
9/21	217	1155
9/22	216	1286
9/23	215.5	1171
9/24	214	1264
9/25	213.5	1130
9/26	212.5	1185

She lost 4 lbs. in one week with true and accurate numbers staying around 1200 calories/day!

~~*~*~*~*~*

This is how I discovered my self-control. With every decision I was free to make, with every calorie I counted and kept track of...

I was in control. Of myself.

Now my roots were growing stronger and deeper. Giant oaks have some of the strongest, deepest roots. With this kind of strength in self-control, a giant oak is not a tree that's easily going to come down through any storm.

Journaling Worksheet

You get to decide what you want to do to create your weight loss. This is step 6. Self-Control. WHERE do you control things? In your journal.

1. A word or two that describes how I feel right now:

2. My weight today:

3. Where do you fall for the recommended number of calories per day for weight loss?

4. Suggested target calories:

    - Up to 150 lbs.: 1200 calories/day
    - 150-250 lbs.: 1200-1400 calories/day
    - 250-350 lbs.: 1400-1800 calories/day
    - 350-450 lbs.: 1800-2400 calories/day.

5. Do you like a limit or a range for your calories?

6. What daily limit or range do you want to set for yourself?

7. For weight loss, does it matter what you eat?

8. Does it matter when you eat?

9. Does it matter how you eat?

10. Does it matter where you eat?

11. Does it matter with who you eat?

12. What is the ONLY thing that creates weight loss?

13. WHERE do you get to control it?

Remember, if you want personal, inspirational, non-judgmental support from Shelley, join Shelley's Club now. She can help. It's this way… www.losingcoach.com.

Step 7 - GRACE

Perfection Not Required!

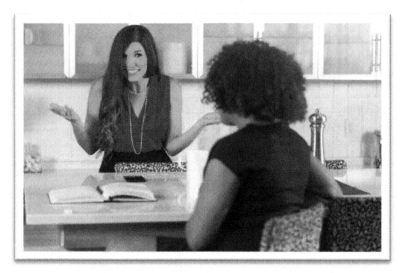

R emoving judgement = GRACE.

The principle of GRACE is found in many religions, doctrines, and ideologies. But NEWSFLASH! (revelation here :)) There is NO GRACE in the universal truth of math.

Repeat—there is NO GRACE in math!

2+2.1 = 4.1

It will never equal 4.

See...there is absolutely no grace in math.

The Losing Coach process respects math 100% of the time.

Because weight loss is *only* attained through math.

So...it is *vital* to have GRACE for, and give GRACE to, ourselves.

Do you consider yourself a gracious person?

To be gracious is to have GRACE.

Do you forgive, act kindly, give people the benefit of the doubt, not hold them in contempt, etc.? Do you consider yourself a non-judgmental person towards others? Great! You understand the concept of GRACE.

Now it's time to give it to yourself.

In this process, we apply GRACE to EVERYTHING, across the board, in all ways and on a day-to-day, minute-by-minute basis:

From understanding your weight gain is not your fault (it's not a character issue).

To the decisions you make on what to eat (nothing is forbidden).

To having a high calorie day (perfection not required).

To a more personal healing of deep wounds from the past (tragic loss, mistreatment).

GRACE is how you <u>LOVE</u> yourself.

The all-encompassing, universal principle of GRACE is what the WHOLE process of permanent weight loss is about.

You can take that huge sigh of relief now. It's okay, even necessary, to apply grace to yourself!

Removing Judgement

Ask yourself this question—are you holding yourself in contempt in any way? The slightest thought of holding yourself in contempt for the loss, for the pain, for the suffering that you've experienced? You may not even realize you are.

I'll just share my own personal story, and again, you can answer it for yourself, okay? Because I don't want you to experience that pain and suffering again. I want to take it off of you. I want you to take it off of yourself. I want you to lift the judgement off.

When I was 25 years old, I gave birth to an extremely premature baby who spent six weeks in the NICU in an incubator. He was developmentally delayed in everything. He was otherwise healthy, for which I was very grateful.

Then, at five years old, he was diagnosed with Tourette's Syndrome, ADHD, and Oppositional Defiance Disorder. But it was the Tourette's Syndrome... I mean, everyone's got ADHD, so that's no big deal. The ODD just meant he was defiant. But it was the Tourette's Syndrome. He's got tics. He's different. He's going to have a difficult time in this life. He's even at higher risk for suicide because of it.

He now is burdened with all of these things. Why? Well, because in my mind anyways, *I* gave birth to him prematurely. Because *I* couldn't carry him.

Sit with that for a moment. My son's life was, in many ways, at risk, for all kinds of heartache and suffering and I felt it was *all* my fault. Do you see how deep a mother's wound is?

People could say all day long, "No, no, no, Shelley, it's not your fault. It's not your fault (your body couldn't carry your baby). These things happen. You couldn't control this. You couldn't have done anything."

You know what? My brain hears you, my logic understands you, and you can tell me this all day long, thank you, but you'll never convince my heart!

You see the judgement and contempt I was holding myself in? Do you feel the heaviness and the pain, and sorrow?

I want you to think about where you've absorbed judgement. Sometimes it's hard to find, and it's hard to recognize, but I want to you think about it. Where is it that you say, 'Thank you, my brain understands I didn't do anything wrong, but... you'll never convince my heart"?

There are lots of ways that we're still holding ourselves in contempt for that loss, that pain and that suffering, my own suffering, or someone else's suffering, that says "I did something wrong."

My mothering energy was deeply wounded. And what is the mothering energy? Remember the LOVE exercise? It was manifested in whomever you gave care, comfort, provision or protection to? Whether to your baby or a parent or a pet, this is the mothering energy inside of you. This is the energy we need healed.

This mothering energy is the energy that we need to tap into.

This is the LOVE energy we need, to power ourselves, and now, we're finding that this LOVE, our mothering energy, has been deeply wounded. And so, we need to validate that wound to take care of that.

Validate your wound, so you can take care of it!

If you come in here with a deep cut and a deep wound, and I say, "Ah, you'll be okay. It's not that big of a deal." And I don't validate how deep your wound is, guess what's going to happen?

No one will take care of it, it's going to get infected, and you're going to lose a limb.

That's why we validate the suffering, so we can tend to it and take care of it and *heal* the wound.

I hope that sums it up and gives you a picture of why we need to validate our suffering. It's not about ruminating in the past, it's about moving forward from it.

(Pointing to her BEFORE photo) Because as soon as I validated her suffering, and had compassion for *her*, something changed ... and she said (whispering) "Thank you...thank you... now someone understands what I've been through."

"That's all I needed, thank you."

Then, she was able to pick herself up, and do what she needed to do, to protect herself. At that moment in time, she needed to lose weight!

And so, she did what she had to do to lose weight. That was her protecting herself. That was her healing the wound.

Here's how I explained removing judgement to my client who was a former stripper.

~~*~*~*~*~*

Shelley: From the little that you've told me, and I'm sure there's more, you've been through a lot. You've been mistreated, and that actually is the reason that you gained weight, from the mistreatment. We'll talk about that later and take that off of you.

It gives me an idea of the fluctuation that your weight has taken, some of the body image things. I mean, even with being a stripper... you were looking for validation. I mean, it gave you validation! You got the attention, the money. That's validation.

Your weight is not a character issue, okay? You are a good person, and you haven't done anything wrong! Nothing.

So, listen to my words, very carefully. You have done nothing wrong. The only reason you were overweight at all is, one-pound equals 3,500 calories, and you've accumulated a surplus of calories over time, that you were unaware of! That's the only reason. It's that simple.

Your need for comfort, which resulted from your painful experiences, created an increased appetite.

Your body knows. Your body knows that it needs comfort, and your body knows that comfort comes from high fat and high sugar foods. You made the judgement that it was a *bad* thing for you to do. It's not. It comforted you, that's your body speaking truth to you. "Something high in fat and high sugar is going to make me feel better, and comfort me right now, after I've been through some distressful experience."

Client: You can call it torture, I call it torture.

Shelley: Yeah. So, torture. So, it spoke truth to you. You attached the judgement to it that you've done something wrong.

You attached judgement and then you compounded it. You attached the judgement: "I'm going to eat something *bad* right now, and I'm *bad* now for wanting to eat something *bad*."
Remove that judgement. Of course, you wanted something that was higher in fat, and higher in sugar, because that would have given you a more instant comfort. That's the truth about food right there. High fat, high sugar foods give more comfort than a bag of cauliflower.

Client: Yeah.

Shelley: So, there is truth in what your body was communicating to you. Don't judge it.

Client: I don't know why I do that.

Shelley: Well, don't judge yourself for it. I want you to know, I don't judge you for judging, either! I'm not judging you for judging. (laughing)

This is not a religious program, but it really is the same message of the Christ. I use Biblical stories, not to tell you where you should place your faith, but because they nicely illuminate some wonderful universal principles.

Have you heard the story of Jesus and the lame man who couldn't walk? The lame man reached out for Jesus's cloak to touch him, and said, "What must I do to be saved?"

Jesus said, "Your sins are forgiven. Stand up and walk home. Take your mat and walk home." And he did!

He needed the *removal* of sin, to be able to do that. He needed the removal of *judgement*. Jesus didn't need to teach him how to walk. Jesus just said, "Your sins are forgiven. Take up your mat and walk home!"

And as soon as he removed the judgement, the man had the ability to walk. Same thing here. I told you last week, in your first coaching session, you hadn't done anything wrong. I told you, in different words, "Your sins are forgiven. Take up your mat, and walk home," and you did!

You have the faith of that man. You exercised the exact same faith the lame man exercised. He believed, accepted, and received. He took up his mat and walked home! You did the same thing! I don't know if you've realized it. You exercised the same amount of *faith* that that man did!

This is not about Jesus' supernatural power and whether you believe in it or not. This is about the principle the story communicates. This is about **GRACE**. This is about *removing judgement* off of you!

~~*~*~*~*~*

Grace is about taking off judgement, so you can walk home.

Home is where all feels right. It feels natural, like you've never done anything wrong. You've returned to your place of origin, who you were always meant to be. Home. It's beautiful. It's the luscious field of green and gold by the riverbank.

Removing Judgement Worksheet

This is Step 7. Grace. The WHOLE thing.

1. A word or two that describes how I feel right now:

2. My weight today:

3. Can you identify a deep wound from the past (mistreatment or tragic event) that you are still holding yourself in contempt for in some way? Are you holding any doubt and/or self-judgement in your heart?

4. Can you lift that contempt/judgement off of yourself, give yourself some tender loving care and allow healing to begin?

5. Is your weight gain your fault? No.

6. Is your weight gain a character issue? No.

7. Is there any morality in math? No.

8. What enabled the lame man to walk?

9. GRACE is what brings the WHOLE process of weight loss mastery together.

   GRACE is what makes the WHOLE process work.

   GRACE makes you WHOLE.

   Can I get an Amen? :)

Remember, if you want personal, inspirational, non-judgmental support from Shelley, join Shelley's Club now. She can help. It's this way... www.losingcoach.com

Seven Simple Steps

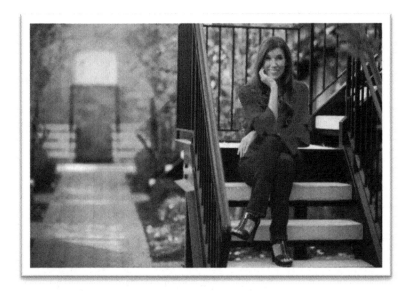

Y ou are through the foundation of the process. Now let's review those seven steps and tie them all together.

This will give you confidence.

Now you can be confident about your weight loss because you have everything you need.

The process is complete.

Spiritually, the number 7 is known as the number of divine completion. There are 7 days in a week, 7 colors in the rainbow, 7 seas and 7 continents.

The Losing Coach process is indeed a complete process, because when all seven steps are put into practice, successful and permanent weight loss is guaranteed.

As you have learned, this is a holistic process.

Here you will see a chart that maps out all seven steps in one place. This will be an anchor point for your future. Remembering and using these seven simple steps will enable you to always weigh what you want to weigh. How do I know? I'll explain in this chapter.

As you read the chapter, remember what you have done and learned already about the Seven Steps.

Seven Simple Steps

Now we're gonna go over the seven steps.

Step 1, Power.

And this was the HOW. *How* are you going to do this? Decision-making, about delay! What we did was known as my "hunger exercise", the acceptance of feeling hungry to delay for your greater purpose.

Step 2, The Simple Truth.

Truth is the math. This is the WHAT.

Step 3, Love.

That is the WHY. That's the mothering energy. Becoming your own mother, giving yourself LOVE to Care, Comfort, Provide and Protect yourself.

Step 4, Faith.

And this is the WHO. This is YOU and your Higher Power for your greater purpose.

Step 5, Hope.

This is the WHEN. And these are your short-term goals.

Step 6, Self-Control.

The physical WHERE of where you are exercising your self-control is in your journal.

Every time that you're looking at calories, measuring things, looking things up, writing it down in your journal, you are exercising self-control!

Step 7, Grace.

This is the WHOLE thing! It's all about this! Perfection not required.

These are the seven steps: Power, Truth, LOVE, Faith, Hope, Self-Control and Grace.

1	Power	How	Decision-Making/Delay
2	Truth	What	The Simple Math
3	LOVE	Why	Mothering Energy - to Care, Comfort, Provide & Protect
4	Faith	Who	YOU & your Higher Power, Your Greater Purpose
5	Hope	When	Short Term Goals
6	Self-Control	Where	Journaling
7	Grace	Whole	Perfection Not Required

So, as you go through your journey of losing weight, week by week, and if you start to struggle, if you start to wonder what's happening, why am I not losing weight as successfully as when I first began? I want you to go to this, these steps, and ask yourself: What is it that I need to focus on this week?

What are my strengths and my weaknesses?

For an example, I'll go through these 7 steps for myself right now. And I'll be really honest on the things that are easy for me and the things that are more challenging for me, the things I need to focus on if I need help losing weight.

Step 1. Power. That actually has become, over the years, *very* easy for me to do. I have no anxiety about delaying my eating. I know I'm going to eat later. This one is now effortless for me!

Step 2. Truth. The math, this is the one that I struggle with more than people would ever realize. As much as I preach about the math, I'm the one that's like, "I think I can eat this and sneak it and get away with it, and my body won't know!" Right?

I forget about the truth of the math, that my body is going to process *everything* that I eat. And so sometimes, for me, if I struggle with managing my weight, I have to remind myself of the truth of the math, that I *can't* get away with things and fool my body; I have to remind myself it will process everything!

Step 3. LOVE. This is actually a great strength of mine now. It was my greatest weakness before but became my greatest strength. This is actually the most challenging for most of my clients... giving themselves this mother's LOVE. That is really the most challenging step, for most women, to give LOVE to themselves.

Step 4. Faith—your letter to God. Go back and read that whenever you need reminded of your purpose, your greater purpose to your greater purpose. What's the meaning behind this weight loss? What's it all for? And who is it between? This is a solid one for me; I'm solid on my faith. If you need reminded, go back and read your letter to God again.

Step 5. Hope. I love this one too, not difficult for me, because I love making charts, and writing numbers, and having hope for the future, and that vision of where I can be in just a week or so.

Step 6. Self-control. This is one that I need to be reminded of, along with Truth, that I have to come back to when I want to manage my weight. I have to say, "Okay. Go back to journaling."

Step 7. Grace. And grace, I'm pretty good at too. I easily remove judgement now. I understand perfection is not required.

So, I know my strengths and weaknesses when it comes to these 7 steps. And if I need help losing weight, I have to ask myself, "Okay, what do I need to focus on?" And usually for me it's these two (truth and self-control). For a lot of women, it's LOVE. Some women struggle with power.

I think that's the first initial thing that people struggle with, the panic of having to delay their gratification. But you practice it and you keep doing it, and this is a muscle that will easily be soon developed. You will realize there's nothing to panic about.

Keep on keeping on and all 7 Steps will become easier and easier.

~~*~*~*~*~*

Is the path really this easy? Well… I'll say it's simple. It's also safe. You have to stay on the path and follow the process. Rest when you need, but stay on the path. It's the escape path out of obesity.

I had to get out of the prison camp.

I stopped listening to all the voices.

I made my escape in privacy.

I accepted I couldn't control certain things like the weather.

I asked for help.

I embraced the fact that the journey was going to take time.

I was empowered to make all my decisions, because I had the power all along.

I stood on the solid ground of truth.

I let LOVE be restored by removing the judgement and receiving the seed of LOVE.

I expressed my faith and my purpose.

I kept reaching.

My roots were strengthened and deepened.

And before I knew it, in this luscious field of green and gold by the riverbank, stood a giant oak, with strong and deep roots. One that had weathered many storms but was still standing. A tree of life.

For a lifetime.

Seven Simple Steps Worksheet

A word or two to describe how I feel right now:

1. My weight today:

2. I have learned about these steps -

3. Power—The HOW. It's all about DELAY.

4. Truth—The WHAT. It's all about the MATH.

5. LOVE—The WHY. It's all about Giving MOTHERING ENERGY to Your Higher Purpose.

6. Faith—The WHO. It's all about You and Your Greater Purpose.

7. Hope—The WHEN. It's all about GOALS.

8. Self-Control. The WHERE. It's all about JOURNALING.

9. Grace. The WHOLE. It's all about PERFECTION-NOT-REQUIRED.

10. The steps I am most confident in and why:

11. The steps that are more challenging to me and why:

And if you need more guidance or encouragement, Shelley's always here with personal, inspirational, non-judgmental support.

Join Shelley's Club now. She can help. It's this way... www.losingcoach.com

EPILOGUE

Last words of advice…

It's so simple, really. Yet it's an entire holistic process that is intertwined and connected to *everything* about you. No pat answer. It's a path I invite you to stay the course on now.

It will take you to your field of green and gold. So, by the riverbank, you can receive the seed of LOVE and become a tree of life.

This is truly for a lifetime.

This is about restoring your dignity. I've learned if you restore a woman's dignity, it's amazing what she can do with her body.

This truth restores a woman's dignity with respect for her, her heart, and her brain. Your privacy restores your dignity. You're able to hear your own thoughts and feel your own feelings and make decisions for yourself.

In some ways, this is teaching you how to diet like a man. Oh, that's right. This is the first time I've mentioned men here. But men are much less likely to hold themselves in contempt for their weight. They don't buy into gimmicks as much, and approach this less emotionally and more practically.

Men love my process. When my clients have gone home and shared with their husbands what this is all about (specifically with respecting the math), husbands reply, "That's what I've been trying to tell you all along!"

It's a cold, harsh truth (eat less, decrease your calories), and you may not have been able to receive it until now. When truth is so cold and harsh, its message can only be received when communicated in LOVE.

The diet industry cannot and will not tell you the truth because it's a multi-billion-dollar industry, with the bottom line being the bottom dollar. So, if it's not marketable, they're not selling it to you. And the *truth is not marketable!* It's available to everyone and nobody owns it. So, they can't sell it.

But now you know the truth.

You possess all seven steps on this path already - Power, Truth, LOVE, Faith, Hope, Self-Control, and Grace. They are YOURS. They are inside you already.

Make your escape. Walk this path. Reach the field. Stand on solid ground. Receive the seed of LOVE. Keep reaching. Let your roots grow deep and strong. Become a giant oak. Be a tree of life.

This is for a lifetime! For the rest of your life, you know how to lose weight

.

ACKNOWLEDGMENTS

I'd like to acknowledge all who are behind this book.

Michele Brenner is the wonderful lady behind getting this book out there; she came to me one day and said, "I can help you publish a book." I said, "Okay!" And she did, and so now this book is in your hands.

Thank you to Erin O'Donnell for documenting her journey through my process to share with the world. I am forever grateful.

Thank you to every Losing Coach client, from my private coaching clients, to workshop participants, to online Shelley's Club members. Every single one of them give me my purpose here and have inspired all my thoughts, ideas, and coaching content, through real, live coaching, communication, and interaction with them.

Thank you to my husband; as I pursued starting a business, he faithfully continued to provide for me and our family.

Thank you to my mom and dad for their unwavering LOVE and support.

Thank you to Neil, Daniel and Luke, my children. They are *my* life's greatest teachers, the ones who taught me how powerful a mother's LOVE is.

And finally, I acknowledge my seed of LOVE, behind absolutely everything I am.

ABOUT THE AUTHOR

S helley was born in Columbus, Ohio and grew up in Worthington, Ohio with her parents, two sisters, and one brother.

When she was seventeen and eighteen, she travelled to Brazil for two summers in a row on mission trips with her youth group. International travelling had officially begun to shape her world view and love for people all over the world.

When she was nineteen, Shelley travelled to Africa on a mission trip with a group of college students from Grace College.

She attended Grace College in Winona Lake, Indiana and earned a Bachelor of Science in Communications.

After college, Shelley lived in Taiwan for a year and taught English as a Second Language. She also travelled to Thailand and Hong Kong.

She then returned to the states, soon got married and began her family.

As a young mother, Shelley mostly stayed at home to raise her sons, but continued to teach and tutor English as a Second Language for a number of years.

In 2001, she began investing in real estate. In 2003, she got her real estate license and became a Realtor.

In January 2006, Shelley began her weight loss journey. By August 2006, she had lost 50 lbs., and came to know her seed of LOVE. By October 2007, Shelley had lost a total of 90 lbs.

Shelley's Before & After photos were published in *Oxygen Magazine* which led her to pursue modeling. She signed with a professional talent agency and began acting and modeling in films and commercials.

Her Before & After photos were published in numerous other magazines, including *Woman's Day*, *Good Housekeeping*, and *Redbook*, and her story was featured in New York Times Best-Seller, Your Best Body Now by Tosca Reno.

In the summer of 2010, Shelley was delegated Mrs. Dublin, Ohio 2010, and competed as a state finalist in the Mrs. Ohio, America pageant. She received the Mrs. Ohio 2010 Career Achievement Award.

She began to coach women by creating and founding The Losing Coach that same summer in 2010.

She has been voted into the Reader's Choice Top 50 Online Weight Loss Coaches in the world.

She has coached many successful, high-profile women, including celebrities, doctors, therapists, business owners, actresses, and models, all to successful weight loss.

Shelley enjoys spending time with her sons, who are now adults, while continuing to coach women all over the world, using her process, to successful weight loss.

Made in the USA
San Bernardino, CA
18 January 2020

63345196R00117